Palgrave Studies in Cyberpsychology

Series Editor
Jens Binder
Nottingham Trent University
Nottingham, UK

Palgrave Studies in Cyberpsychology aims to foster and to chart the scope of research driven by a psychological understanding of the effects of the 'new technology' that is shaping our world after the digital revolution. The series takes an inclusive approach and considers all aspects of human behaviours and experiential states in relation to digital technologies, to the Internet, and to virtual environments. As such, Cyberpsychology reaches out to several neighbouring disciplines, from Human-Computer Interaction to Media and Communication Studies. A core question underpinning the series concerns the actual psychological novelty of new technology. To what extent do we need to expand conventional theories and models to account for cyberpsychological phenomena? At which points is the ubiquitous digitisation of our everyday lives shifting the focus of research questions and research needs? Where do we see implications for our psychological functioning that are likely to outlast short-lived fashions in technology use?

Michael C Nagel • Rachael Sharman

Virtual Autism and Other Screen Disorders

palgrave
macmillan

Michael C Nagel
Child and Adolescent Development
University of the Sunshine Coast
Queensland, QLD, Australia

Rachael Sharman
School of Health
University of the Sunshine Coast
Queensland, QLD, Australia

ISSN 2946-2754 ISSN 2946-2762 (electronic)
Palgrave Studies in Cyberpsychology
ISBN 978-3-032-00802-2 ISBN 978-3-032-00803-9 (eBook)
https://doi.org/10.1007/978-3-032-00803-9

This Palgrave Macmillan imprint is published by the registered company Springer Nature Switzerland AG.
The registered company address is: Gewerbestrasse 11, 6330 Cham, Switzerland

This book is dedicated to parents, teachers and all those who support children and teens as they orientate themselves and grow into adulthood.

Preface

What's Happening to Young Minds?

The times they are a changin'! In 1964 Bob Dylan released that song as the title track of his album of the same name. That song has been interpreted a number of ways but its central premise focuses on how people view society. In terms of child and adolescent development, we think how people view society is arguably more pertinent now than any other time in human history. And although we, the authors, were born at different times, one a Baby Boomer and the other a Gen Xer, our current views on society and the years in which we grew from children to adults were remarkably similar. We can recall a time when our telephones were not mobile and usually fastened to the wall somewhere in our homes. Televisions were not flat but instead were often one of the largest pieces of furniture in the living room with less than vibrant sound and where colour images were a luxury. Our news was never described as 'fake' and was only available at certain times of the day. If something happened on the other side of the world we did not hear about it in real time and rarely would breaking news interfere with the myriad of TV game shows where the grand prize might be a car if one was lucky. We played games on boards not on screens and more often than not we were told to go outside and play until it got dark.

We are not wanting to appear overly sentimental or romanticising the past. We are only trying to highlight how things have changed so very much in such a very short time for generations living in the twenty-first century. The things we read about in science fiction books or saw in the same genre of movies are now part of our lives and we take them for granted. We have access to the world in the palm of our hands and live at a time when the boundaries between what defines us as humans in comparison to the technology we use are becoming increasingly blurred. Indeed, technology continues to make ever greater inroads into our lives, however, we question whether this is always a good thing? In order to understand our thinking, we invite you to consider that technological inroads may actually be intrusions and altering the brains and minds of twenty-first-century young people in ways we are only beginning to understand. Invoking some lines from Dylan's song we would contend that, *the battle outside ragin', will soon shake your windows and rattle your walls, for the times they are a changin'.*

The claims above may appear alarming and they are intended to, given the research we have looked at is inherently alarming. However, before we start to share this evidence and unpack how technology is impacting on the brains and minds of today's youth we would like to make two important points for consideration.

First, we are not Luddites! Some who have read our bodies of work or heard us speak at conferences or via various media platforms have been quick to proclaim that we like to romanticise about the past and are looking to turn back time. Let us be clear, we like our screens and use them regularly! We watch TV, do online shopping and often chat with friends and family in far-away places via online platforms. Much of our work requires us to use technology and the pages you are reading now were not transcribed from stone tablets. We work in an information economy and we embrace technology for all it offers but we do think using screen devices should be a cautionary tale for all, and especially for those whose brains are still developing.

Second, any talk of human dysfunction and disorder can attract calls of "ableist" from those uncomfortable discussing difficult topics. An ableist is someone who, through a sense of superiority, defines a person by their disability and/or discriminates against people with disabilities and/

or views disabilities as something to be fixed. We do not define anyone by their abilities or lack thereof, nor would we label anyone beyond what we see in the scientific literature. Phrases like 'virtual autism' may be uncomfortable for some but those feelings do not diminish the presence of that phenomenon—a presence that is increasingly prescient in clinical and scientific research.

It is also interesting that while some might bemoan the use of particular phrases or labels, they are perfectly comfortable with attaching their own labels to others. Labels are easy to fling around at people whose views you may not share. We see this as part of a problem that we actually unravel in this book. We live in a time when those who will not, or cannot, see things from another perspective, something known as 'theory of mind', attack the person or persons instead of arguing against their arguments or ideas. Attacking a person rather than discussing and debating their position is both easy and lazy and hardly ever worth responding to, so we don't. We will let you, the reader, make your own decisions.

Now, back to the foundation of this book and our central premise around the impact of screens on young minds. Let's begin by recognising that since the turn of the century there has been a great deal of medical and scientific research in most things to do with the brain. Much of this research has focused on the impact of technology and screen devices on child and adolescent brain development at the nexus of understanding overall development. Everything from cognitive processing to concentration to attention to physical health and psychological wellbeing have come under the curious eyes of researchers. This is of particular interest to those with concerns related to the potential impact of a 'screen-driven' culture and society on the minds and bodies of a species whose brain takes almost 30 years to fully mature. Yes, you read correctly. The human brain is not fully developed until sometime after our 24th birthday depending on whether you are male or female. Most of the hard work related to maturation is done by the time we turn 20 with some fine-tuning taking place for a few more years. What this means is that some of the most crucial aspects of brain development occur in children and teenagers. Significantly, this development occurs in a world vastly different from previous generations.

We noted earlier that the times are a changin'. Humanity has experienced many technological innovations over time but at no time in history has information and technology had such a pervasive impact on all that we experience and by association on all aspects of human development. Moreover, and as each day passes, it is evident that the influence of screen devices is only increasing. This is particularly significant when we consider what constitutes healthy development for children and teens.

As researchers our curiosity and interests expand across a range of developmental considerations and as such we think that the interplay between young people and technology is worth a great deal of scrutiny. We also think it important to alert parents and teachers to the increasingly troubling dark side of screen use given their role in nurturing young minds. This book is a sincere attempt to do just that—give insights and advice regarding screen use and the developing brain.

In writing this book it was never our intention to ask people to abandon screens. We think such reductionist thinking is not realistic; we are not ever going to go backwards as that is not human nature. We would argue, however, that the burgeoning number of studies linked to potential negative outcomes associated with screen usage should give us pause to think. This thinking would do well to adopt a 'cautionary' mindset. It is time to examine the breadth of research looking at the risks associated with screen usage and time on screens and be cautious in circumstances when there is a great deal of uncertainty, especially when the risks might be exceedingly high. This is something we unpack throughout this book and as such there are things that have shaped our perspectives that should be noted here.

First, we would contend that too much of the discussion around screen devices, social media, gaming, other forms of tech use and young people is dominated by individuals and/or organisations with a vested interest in promoting the use of technology. For example, media experts, 'e-learning' (electronic learning) advocates and/or politicians will often offer soundbites of authority suggesting technology is a panacea for life and learning and necessary for higher educational standards. The problem here should be obvious...their expertise is not in child and adolescent development or health.

Second, any discussion of screens, children and teens must look long and hard at what young people are consuming. The content young people are absorbing, and the experiences they are having on screen devices is deeply worrying. Access to violence, pornography and other troubling aspects of content coupled with the anonymity inherent in any social media platforms means that children and teens are simply left vulnerable to less than positive influences. This vulnerability exists 24/7 and unlike previous generations cannot be curtailed simply by being at home or school and under the watchful gaze of parents and teachers. Being sent to one's room in the twenty-first century is not always done in isolation where the constant opportunity for unfettered access to 'friends', being 'liked', creating videos or being an influencer can happen anywhere and at any time.

Finally, and related to the points above, those who work in the areas of child development, psychology and neuroscience are not simply concerned with technology and content per se or hold any sense of being 'anti-technology' as alluded to earlier. What is troubling to us is a lack of mainstream understanding regarding the premature use or overuse of screens by young people whose brains and bodies are not yet fully formed coupled with an increasing number of studies saying that all is not right when kids spend time on devices. The pervasive nature of screens along with the taken-for-granted ubiquity of screen devices appears to be having a deleterious effect on developing brains. Therefore, it is our contention that screen time must be considered a major public health issue and reducing screen time must become the new priority for child and adolescent health. This is particularly evident in the stories and examples provided in the chapters you are about to read.

Queensland, QLD, Australia — Michael C. Nagel
Queensland, QLD, Australia — Rachael Sharman

Competing Interests The authors have no competing interests to declare that are relevant to the content of this manuscript.

About the Book

This book explores the pervasive impact of technology on the developing brains of young people. For example, there is a growing body of research documenting 'autistic'-like behaviours in children and adolescents as a function of their exposure to screen-based technologies. Furthermore, and given the omnipotence of online social platforms in increasingly more aspects of day-to-day lives, it is important that society understands the generational impacts of brain changes, and by association potential behavioural manifestations in response to screen-based social platforms. Questions need to be raised regarding the trajectory of future generations that may include underdeveloped aspects of interpersonal social skills, and the impact of this on those who will potentially go on to reshape the social norms and expectations of society.

Contents

About the Authors

Michael C Nagel and Rachael Sharman are first and foremost parents with many years of experience navigating that space. Being parents is one of the factors that motivated them to put this volume together. Being scholars and academics, however, was the principal driver for sharing their expertise and ideas in this field. Their shared interest in child and adolescent development has nurtured collaborations across a range of articles, presentations and books and is evident in their biographies. Aside from being Co-Editors for *The Encyclopedia of Child and Adolescent Development* Drs Nagel and Sharman have also contributed to our understanding of child and adolescent development across numerous platforms and audiences.

Michael C Nagel is an Associate Professor at the University of the Sunshine Coast and teaches and researches in the areas of child and adolescent development, behaviour and learning. He has authored 23 books focusing broadly on aspects of educational psychology and child development. His books are housed and used by students in libraries across more than 40 countries and in numerous universities including, but not limited to, University of California at Berkeley, Harvard, Oxford, Stanford, The Washington Library of Congress, University College London, Columbia University and Johns Hopkins University. Aside from his teaching and research activity Dr Nagel has delivered more than 100 keynote addresses and has conducted workshops and seminars for teachers and parents at over 300 schools in Australia and abroad. He has been an invited guest on 'TV New Zealand Breakfast', 'Sunrise', ABC National and 'The Project'. Dr Nagel has been a feature writer for the 'The First Five Years' online parenting platform and for 'Jigsaw' and the 'Child' series of magazines which collectively offers parenting advice to more than one million parents.

Rachael Sharman is Senior Lecturer and researcher in Psychology at the University of the Sunshine Coast, specialising in child and adolescent development. Dr Sharman's research is focused on the optimal and healthy development of the paediatric brain and she has published over 30 peer-reviewed journal articles, two book chapters and one co-authored book.

Prior to her career in academia, Dr Sharman worked for over 15 years in a variety of child-related fields including child protection, juvenile justice (forensics), disability, advocacy and genetic research. In 2002, she successfully lobbied the Queensland Government to invest in expanded newborn screening. This has prevented the unnecessary death or disability caused by rare genetic disorders if left undetected and untreated. Dr Sharman is also an enthusiastic and engaging public speaker with a weekly ABC radio guest appearance, and a variety of media published in newspapers, magazines (Time), internet (ABC, The Conversation) and television (news, The Project, SBS Insight).

List of Figures

1

Not a Blank Slate…

Our species has successfully taken over every corner of the globe because we represent the highest expression of a trick that Mother Nature discovered: don't entirely pre-script the brain; instead, just set it up with the basic building blocks and get it into the world.
—Dr David Eagleman (2020, p. 3)

Abstract This chapter explores the remarkable complexity and plasticity of the human brain, describing how it develops from birth through adulthood. The brain contains trillions of neural connections—with one cubic millimetre storing approximately two thousand terabytes of data—and forms these connections through environmental experiences. The chapter examines key brain structures (brain stem, limbic system, and cerebrum) and their functions, highlighting the frontal lobes as the "CEO" of the brain which don't fully mature until around age 25. Two critical developmental processes are explained: "experience-expectant" stimulation (universal processes like vision development) and "experience-dependent" stimulation (individualised learning shaped by environment). The chapter also documents aspects of the brain's neuroplasticity—its ability to reorganise itself—which is particularly powerful during childhood and

M. C. Nagel, R. Sharman, *Virtual Autism and Other Screen Disorders*, Palgrave Studies in Cyberpsychology, https://doi.org/10.1007/978-3-032-00803-9_1

adolescence but diminishes with age. This understanding of brain development provides crucial context for understanding how environmental factors, including screen use, can shape neural pathways and behaviours during formative years.

Keywords Neurons • Synapse • Brain stem • Cerebellum • Limbic system • Cerebrum • Prefrontal cortex • Neuroplasticity

Setting up the basic building blocks of the brain and get it into the world! This is a critical piece of the puzzle we will be building for you in this book; being out in the world shapes the settings of our brain. And while setting the brain up sounds simple enough, understanding the brain is a bit more complex. Neuroscientist and best-selling author, Professor Joseph LeDoux has described the brain as the most unimaginable thing imaginable[1] … and for good reason. Try to wrap your own brain around this … you are walking on a beach and reach down to pick up some sand. With great dexterity you manage to get rid of all the sand but one small grain. If you have the time and inclination to measure that grain of sand you would find it to be about one cubic millimetre. Now consider this, if you were able to hold a piece of the brain that same size, one cubic millimetre, in your hand you would be holding something that stores about two thousand terabytes of data—enough storage space for all the movies ever made including their trailers. Having difficulty thinking about all the movies ever made, well then try this on for size. Two thousand terabytes of data is equivalent to 1.2 billion copies of a 500-page textbook. It has been suggested that the brain, in its entirety, could store 200 exabytes of data which is enough to hold the entire digital content of the world. These astounding facts were published in one of the world's most prestigious neuroscientific journals in 2013 and made news headlines globally and fodder for writers and brain enthusiasts alike.[2]

[1] LeDoux (1998).

[2] The journal and author that published the article on the brain and its memory is Alison Abbott in *Nature Neuroscience*, volume 499 published in July 2013. Bill Bryson very eloquently outlines this and other amazing facts about the brain in his 2019 book entitled *The Body*.

If we wanted, we could go on and list more amazing trivia about the gelatinous mass between your ears, but we think you get the point. Our brains are uniquely special in what they do, how they do it and how they learn to do everything we often take for granted. The brain is never entirely a blank slate. Not long after conception the brain forms and starts to create neural pathways for ensuring our survival and for learning. This learning occurs via our experiences and the nature of those experiences shapes the blueprint of our existence and behaviours. In order to understand how this occurs, it is important to know just a bit about how the brain is structured, how it uses information it receives from the environment and how this works in tandem with its 'plasticity' or capacity to change. So sit back and continue to imagine the unimaginable.

Imagining the Unimaginable

Let's start by simply holding an image of the brain in your mind. Most people might mention its football like shape and its wrinkly looking hemispheres. Chances are, however, that any description by the layperson would not go too far beyond the kind of general description provided above given most people know very little about the very thing that allows them to think, feel and do what they do every day. Truth be told, most neuroscientists would concede that they know very little about the brain in comparison to what they would like to know. Part of the reason, beyond the brain's inherent complexity, is that we have only really had access to its inner workings since just before the turn of the century.

On July 17, 1990, the signing of Presidential Proclamation 6158 by then President of the United States George H.W. Bush provided a global catalyst for an exponential growth of research funding in neuroscience. That proclamation basically labelled the 1990s as the 'Decade of the Brain' with the beginning of the twenty-first century being heralded as the age of brain-mind science.[3] Advances in technology coupled with a growing body of research on, or about, the brain saw numerous professions reinvigorated with insights into how the brain grows, learns

[3] Goldberg (2001).

and operates. Psychologists, therapists, physicians and educators, to name a few, were increasingly armed with a growing understanding of how the brain and mind define us as a species and separate us from all other life forms on the planet. Questions related to mental health, ageing, cognition, memory, learning, emotions, behaviour and general wellbeing were increasingly informed by neuroscience. Brain imaging and research made the language of brain science available to the public at large. People started to joke about faulty synapses and brain fog while the shelves of bookstores exploded with a vast array of works on how to understand and get the best out of our brains. Yet, and despite all the work over the last few decades, there is still so much we don't know. The brain is still rather mysterious but there are some things that are necessary for you to understand in order to see how the building blocks of the brain and mind are shaped by the environment.

First, some basics. About the size of a coconut, a mature brain weighs roughly one and a half kilograms, or three pounds. It is a massive collection of nerve cells. The two prominent types of cells are called glial cells and neurons. Glial cells are important but our interest lies in neurons for this is where all the action is!

Neurons begin to emerge in utero, and at birth the brain actually has more neurons than it needs but little connectivity between them. In its simplest sense, neurons take in information via environmental stimulation and pass that information to where it is needed. For example, as you read these words, your eyes are taking that information and passing it through a superhighway of neural connectivity to your occipital lobes where it is 'seen' and then translated to other parts of the brain involved in language. If you haven't read between the lines, it is not your eyes that see, but rather the lobes at the back of the brain that use the eyes as an instrument for sourcing and translating visual stimulation, or 'seeing' … another amazing bit of brain trivia that sometimes freaks people out.

In the early years of life, roughly from birth to age four, at least one million connections between neurons are made every second. An amazing number and far more than any other time in life. By the time a child reaches their third birthday they will have more neural connections than their paediatrician. During adolescence the brain 'prunes' back some of those connections to become more refined and efficient. That is, the brain actually eliminates connections that are un-used, un-needed or unimportant to survival in that particular environment. That's right dear reader, the process of learning and fine-tuning our brain into adulthood relies on cell-death, not cell growth. The sponges we were as children now refine themselves down to the connections that are required for best operational practice in the environment we live in. We will expand on what happens to the brain during adolescence in greater detail in chapter two but for now remember that establishing the inner wiring of the brain early in life enables a child to control their body and start learning about the world. Later on, the unnecessary connections are discarded so the adolescent can hone their focus and concentrate on what is most important to understand the world around them.

Different areas of the brain are responsible for different things. There are parts that take care of movement, emotion and language. All of these which develop at different rates and their connections grow in complexity. As a child matures in age, so too does the brain and with its expanding neural superhighway it learns to move, speak and think in increasingly complex ways. Think of your child's brain as a developing orchestra. At first practice some sections of the orchestra are too loud, or lagging behind, making for a sometimes frustrating and unpleasant outcome! But finally as practice makes perfect and the conductor (frontal lobes in our analogy) take over, we begin to hear that polished performance.

The trillions of connections begin to form because of something that is happening in the outside world, and in a way neurons speak to each other. The passing of information between neurons actually happens through an electro-chemical impulse and is a process more commonly referred to as synapses. No two neurons in the human brain physically touch, and the impulses noted above rely on a variety of chemical messengers known as neurotransmitters. Dopamine, for example, is a powerful neurotransmitter associated with rewards, sensation seeking and pleasure; all important considerations in terms of screen use. We will expand on connections between screen use and neurotransmitters at different points throughout the book given neurotransmitters' role in shaping how we feel and behave. As a teaser, keep this stored in your memory … screen devices, social media sites and apps are designed with dopamine in mind!

At this juncture we hope you have come to realise that the early stages of life are very important in shaping who we are and who we become. The experiences we have, and the relationships with parents, siblings, loved ones and peers, literally help to lay out the connections in our brains. The importance of experiences is elaborated on later in this chapter but prior to that it is also significant to have some understanding of the basic structures of the brain … a bit more neuroscience for you!

The Architecture of Our Mind

Before looking at specific regions and structures of the brain it is probably worth highlighting that the brain and mind are not the same thing. We sometimes use those words interchangeably, but they are indeed different. When we use the word brain, we are referring to all the structures and physiological processes attended to and mediated by that electrochemical mass inside our skulls. The mind, alternatively, can simply be considered as something the brain does.[4] The mind is a product of the brain and includes a myriad of activities including intelligence, consciousness, learning strategies, the capacity to form language and perhaps most notably, the capacity to think about thinking.[5] In order for the mind to work and do all that it does, it relies on the process of neural connectivity noted earlier along with structures within the brain.

Earlier we noted how people generally have a shared understanding of what the brain looks like and that it has two hemispheres. Those hemispheres are only part of the structural story. There are bits and pieces in different regions of the brain that have specific roles in shaping our thoughts, feelings and behaviours. Those bits and pieces can be found in three principal regions of the brain known as the brain stem, limbic system and cerebrum. We split them into three to discuss their primary functions, but they are intimately connected to one another and collectively allow our minds to engage with the world as necessary.

[4] Pinker (2009).

[5] Nagel (2012).

The brain stem sits at the base of the brain and connects the spinal cord to the brain. The brain stem plays a role in many things including vomiting, sneezing and coughing along with critical functions such as cardiac rhythm, blood pressure and breathing; a neck injury and trauma to the brain stem can be life threatening.[6] The brain stem is also our survival control centre. When our brain declares something as a threat, it is the brain stem that initiates our 'fight-or-flight' response. Without the brain stem operating at its optimum we would not be able to alert our bodies to stand our ground and prepare for battle or take up flight and run for our lives. The brain stem has, from an evolutionary standpoint, ensured our survival. There is however one small drawback with the brain stem. Too often in our modern world we can misinterpret normal day-to-day interactions as threats whereby the brain stem does its job and gets us ready to fight or run away when it really isn't necessary to do so. Historically, our 'fight-or-flight' response used to be something relied upon for short-term purposes so we could avoid actual threats like sabre tooth tigers or not so friendly neighbouring tribes. Arguments, frustration with someone at a service counter, being cut off by an inconsiderate driver or any other manner of contemporary agitations can set of our alarm bells in our brain stem and result in powerful chemicals being poured into our bloodstream which are unnecessary, and long term, can be terribly unhealthy.

Another important structure sitting just above the brain stem and worthy of some mention is the cerebellum. This complex structure houses about 50% of our neurons which is why scientists decided to use the Latin word for 'little brain' when they named it. The list of responsibilities related to the cerebellum or the challenges associated with damage to this structure are far reaching. For the purpose of brevity, it is probably best to remember that the cerebellum not only helps to shape or thoughts and movements but also has a role to play in processing emotions given its connections to the limbic system (Fig. 1.1).

The limbic system, which sits just above the brain stem and cerebellum and in the middle of both hemispheres is our emotional heartland. In its simplest sense, the limbic system is a collection of structures involved in

[6] Nagel and Scholes (2016); see also Carter (2009); Sweeney (2009); D'angelo (2019).

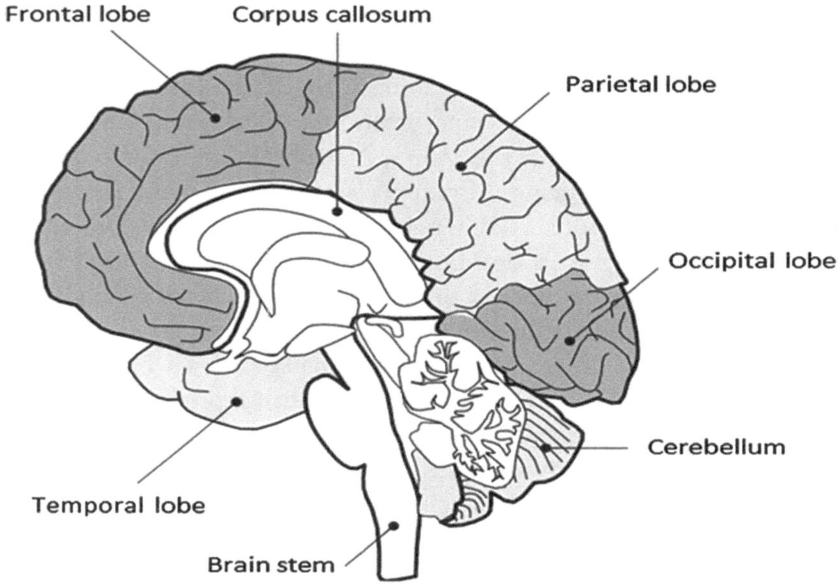

Fig. 1.1 Image of brainstem and cerebellum

all of our emotions and emotional processing along with various aspects of memory. If you were to think of something from your past that generated feelings of happiness, and we were using brain imaging technology to see what is going on inside your heard, we would see parts of your limbic system fast at work. And while emotions and memories are important, the limbic system also has a role to play in motivation, our sleep patterns, hormones, attention, the regulation of bodily functions and many other mechanisms that shape our behaviours. The limbic system also plays a part in influencing many of the higher-order thinking processes that occur in our cerebrum (Fig. 1.2).[7]

For a majority of people, the cerebrum is probably the most familiar part of the brain. It is the largest section, or region of the brain, comprising of two hemispheres that are surrounded by a thin layer of cells called the cerebral cortex. This is the thinking part of the brain and it

[7] Nagel (2012).

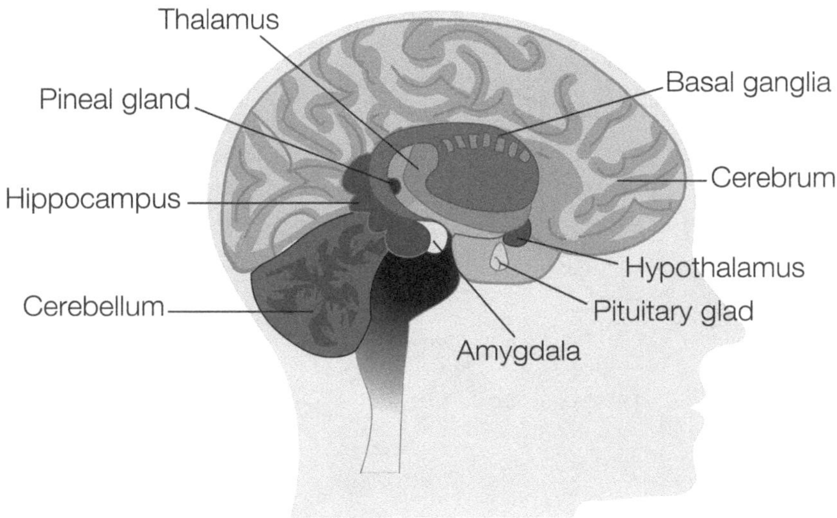

Fig. 1.2 Image of limbic system

consists of four lobes, each with some primary responsibilities. The occipital lobes mentioned earlier in the chapter sit at the back of the brain and process visual information. Roughly speaking, move forward and up from the occipital lobes and you have the parietal lobes that manage sensory information like touch and temperature; move forward and down you find the temporal lobes that manage auditory information and also process some visual stimuli. Within each of those lobes other functions occur. For example, the comprehension and forming of language occurs mainly in the left temporal lobe. And while all of these lobes are important in their own right, they are outmatched by the frontal lobes or what could be referred to as the CEO of the brain (Fig. 1.3).

The frontal lobes are what separates us from the monkeys (well, somewhat)! Our primate cousins have frontal lobes as do other mammals but they are nowhere near as big or complex as ours. The frontal lobes are basically where higher-order thinking occurs. Neuroscientists use the term 'executive functions' to describe all the important things the frontal

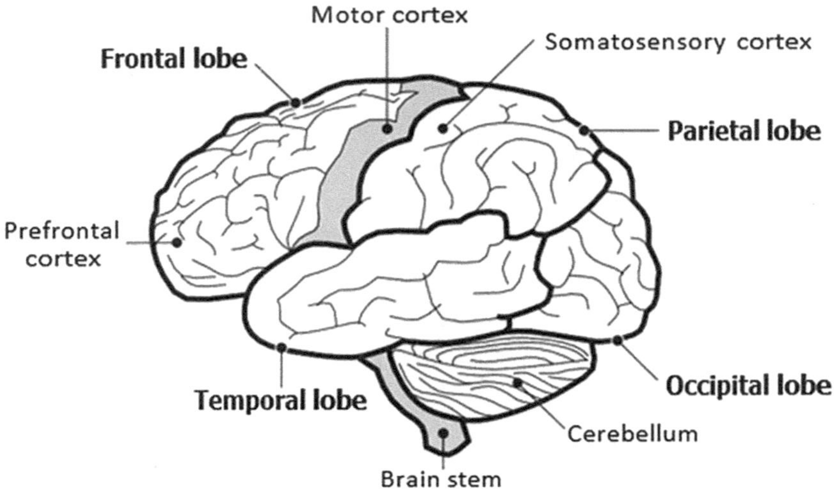

Fig. 1.3 Image of cerebrum

lobes, and in particular the right prefrontal cortex, do. Many of these things we simply take for granted but damage to your frontal lobes could impact on your attention, concentration, planning, emotional regulation, judgement, empathy, and problem-solving and decision-making abilities amongst many other important things and functions. Importantly, the frontal lobes don't fully mature until long past the teenage years.

In computer jargon, our frontal lobes don't fully come 'online' until somewhere around our 25th birthday. It isn't an exact science but it seems that most of the hard work related to brain maturation is complete around 19 years of age with full maturation for females around 24 and males a year or two later. This is why things like controlling our emotions can be challenging for children or why teens might do things that make adults shake their heads in disbelief; the analytical part of the immature brain is often hostage to the survival and emotional regions of the brain. It is also noteworthy that the brain's CEO is continually influenced and potentially shaped by the environment due to its plastic nature.

Experiences Matter!

Recall the opening of this chapter ... with the building blocks set in place, the world shapes our brains. We are prewired to do things but environmental stimulation and experiences lead to our brains becoming hardwired.[8] Experiences matter and literally shape our brains. Not all experiences are the same, however, and nature and nurture work in tandem to sculpt minds and behaviours. Specifically, we rely on 'experience-expectant' stimulation and 'experience-dependent' stimulation to construct our neural pathways and shape who we become.

Consider what would happen if you were deprived of certain experiences early in life. That was the basis of the work of Nobel Prize winning neuroscientists David Hubel and Torsten Wiesel when they sutured shut one eyelid of a number of newborn kittens. The kittens were then allowed to grow into adulthood before the eyelid was reopened. Hubel and Torsten found a stark difference in the functioning of the eyes whereby the sutured eye could not see, even though that eye was undamaged. In essence the kitten was deprived of the stimulation necessary to hardwire for sight.[9] It turns out that there are critical times that the brain 'expects' to have various types of stimulation to hardwire for certain functions. We also know this is the case with infants, not because anyone has ever stitched their eyelids shut, but an infant born with cataracts is at risk of vision impairment lest those cataracts be removed. As adults, if we develop cataracts and delay their removal, once removed our vision returns to where it was pre-cataracts; as we were already prewired for sight.

As human beings all our senses are rather rudimentary at birth and as the brain matures it expects an array of environmental stimuli to help set wiring into place. Relatedly, and barring any physical impairments or extreme deprivation of stimulation, the everyday experiences of life will provide what is needed for much of our neural hardwiring. Remember the brain has its basic building blocks in place and is 'prewired' for certain abilities to unfold. If, on the other hand, a child is deprived of certain experiences due to trauma and/or severe neglect then that child is being

[8] Mitchell (2018).

[9] Hubel and Wiesel (1970).

primed for any number of developmental difficulties including, but not limited to, cognitive deficits, difficulties with attention and concentration, behavioural problems and any number of socio-emotional challenges. We provide examples of this later in chapter six. At this stage it is important to remember that early life experiences, or the lack thereof, create differences in abilities and behaviours. Again, something to keep in mind in any conversation about screens and most notably in the context of experience 'dependent' stimulation.

While the types of experiences discussed above could be referred to as 'nature', experience 'dependent' stimulation would definitely fall under the label of 'nurture'. These are the experiences that are provided to us by the people, circumstances and events in our lives. If you wanted to distill it even further, you could simply call it 'learning'. By way of example think of a parent showing an infant how to hold a spoon for the first time and start feeding themself. As most parents would attest to, initially this can be frustrating and messy for both parent and child. However, over time, and with practice, that infant's brain will develop the neural pathways for all that is required to use the spoon effortlessly and without having to consciously think about the actions of feeding itself.

It should be apparent from the example above that experiences and what adults do to, and with, children matters for a developing brain. The brain is very malleable and 'plastic' in our youth and as such shaped by what happens around it. We will talk about 'plasticity' shortly but prior to doing so, some final considerations related to experiences are worth noting.

First, no two brains are the same and as such simply providing certain experiences will not always result in exactly the same outcomes. There will always be individual variations in development even when the environment is the same so what we are offering here is a broad overview of how experiences in the outer world shape our inner neural environments. The vast majority of parents will tell you that in spite of growing up in the same house, with the same parents and same opportunities, their children can be very different. We all have building blocks to be set up and nurtured but not all blocks are identical. Some of those blocks have different biological and genetic markers which will have some influence on how the environment is actually experienced. If this were not the case then we would not have variations in dominant handedness, personality, learning disabilities or any number of other factors linked to our genes.

Second, while no two brains are the same, nor all experiences, experience-expectant development is a universal process that applies to all children. Provide visual stimulation to an infant in Australia, Peru, Madagascar or any other part of the world and the brain will hardwire for sight. Conversely, and as alluded to above, experience-dependent processes are far more individual and contextual. All children will have the building blocks for language but where they are raised will dictate their native tongue, and indeed the accent they develop.

Finally, while experiences are important and literally help to shape the brain, this doesn't mean that children should be overly inundated with experiences by overzealous parents, caregivers or educators. Neuroscience has given us a great deal of understanding about the developing brain but sometimes it can be used in less than scientific ways. Not long ago, for example, an infomercial broadcast during prime-time television viewing purported that 'brain science' tells us that two-year-olds could learn to read. The myth-information presented suggested that an abundance of early stimulation using flashcards and other tools for reading, with the help of an adult, would set a child up with early linguistic prowess towards untold benefits in school. The problem is the very parts of the brain that allow you to recognise, sound and decipher letters and sounds simple aren't 'online' at two years of age. A child might learn to mimic a 'parroting' adult but mimicry and reading are two very different things. The brain has its own developmental timelines and no amount of hyper-stimulation by increasing the quantity of particular experiences will impact on that timeline. Doing too much too soon however could create measures of anxiety and stress in children with the end result being that more may actually be less. It is the quality of experiences that matters at particular times and not the quantity. As we learn more about the brain perhaps one day we might find a way to build a better brain sooner given the fact that the brain can and does change due to its 'plastic' nature.

The Brain's Ability to Change

Arguably, most people have heard something about brain 'plasticity'. Not long ago, it was believed that the brain was mostly unchangeable. It was described as having a specific number of cells and neural circuits that remained unchanged unless damaged in some way. Scientists have learned, however, that the brain does indeed change and can do so in seconds, over time, or not at all depending on age. This ability to change has become known as 'neuroplasticity' and encompasses the brain's ability to adapt and modify itself in response to environmental stimuli.[10] For example, if your flow of concentration during the reading of this page was suddenly interrupted by the surprising or fearful sound of a loud bang, we could see changes to your neural circuitry. We admit that we would need to be looking at your brain through brain-imaging technology but you get the point—the brain can change, sometimes instantaneously, and does so regularly.

To have a good understanding of the links between the brain and the potential impact of technology on its plastic nature, we think there are a couple of things you should keep in the back of your mind as you move through this chapter and the rest of this book. First and foremost, through childhood and adolescence the brain's primary job is to change itself.[11] Remember that a child's brain has more neural connections than it needs with some getting pruned back during adolescence. And this process of eliminating unused connections is directly linked to experience … what a teen spends time doing strengthens connections while others simply fade away. This is one example of the brain's neuroplasticity, but it is very much one of the most important given the role of the environment in shaping the mind. 'Use it or lose it' is a simple adaptive response to fine-tuning the brain and making it more efficient but what goes in also shapes what comes out.

The amazing, and yet seemingly simple act of 'pruning', described above is not the only thing that is age related. In order to explain this we would like you to think of 'silly putty' and 'cement'.

---

[10] Voss et al. (2017).

[11] Mitchell (2018).

Given the time required for the brain to fully mature it could be noted that the process is more marathon than sprint. The brain is set with the building blocks in place and primed for experience. At birth the brain is very plastic or malleable and is molded, like silly putty, by the myriad of experiences a child encounters and the environment. The more repetitive an experience, or the more something is practised, the firmer the silly putty becomes but it can still be reshaped when puberty takes hold. Over time, however, the silly putty becomes more like cement. That is not a snide commentary on teenagers having concrete in their heads, although some might wonder at times. Instead, it is a precursor to knowing that at some point our plastic brains become less so in terms of how they may or may not change. Some examples of plasticity will help explain the point.

Let's start by thinking of a time when you may have been caught by surprise by a ferociously barking dog. For most people such an encounter would make their heart rates increase, see goosebumps emerge, experience a sweat breaking out and/or a yelp or scream while seemingly jumping out of their skin. At that point in time the brain is busy making a determination, freeze like a statue, prepare for battle or run like hell. All of this decision-making would result in a milieu of measurable changes to the neural architecture of the brain. Turns out that being scared to death, as well as a range of many other emotions, literally changes the brain.

You probably never think of it but meeting new people, practising playing a guitar, watching your favourite TV show or even reading the words you are reading makes a demonstrable change in your neural hardwiring. It might be easier to think of the brain as being something that is continually 'livewired' considering it operates as a "dynamic, adaptable, information seeking system".[12] This is a wet cement version of plasticity but there is a less accommodating form of cement that hardens as we get older.

One of the unfortunate facts of ageing is that a fully developed brain is more susceptible to long-term challenges and difficulties resulting from ill health or injury. As we get older some aspects of our neuroplasticity gain a degree of permanency. A young lady by the name of Jodie Miller offers a great example of what we are now outlining.

[12] Eagleman (2020, p. 14).

Not long after her birth in 1990, Jodie Miller would begin to suffer from a rare condition known as Rasmussen's encephalitis. This very unpleasant neurological disease results in chronic inflammation and can result in severe seizures, loss of motor skills and speech, weakness to one side of the body and dementia-like behaviours. This disease generally occurs in children under the age of 15 and by three years of age the right hemisphere of Jodie's brain was inflamed and she was increasingly experiencing life-threatening seizures. These would lead to complete paralysis in the left side of her body due to the fact that our brains are contralateral—the right hemisphere controls the left side of the body and vice versa.

Imagine, if you can, suddenly losing all control over half of your body. For Jodie her seizures were increasing in frequency and severity and she was not responding to any types of medical interventions so her quality of life was diminishing rapidly. The doctors, therefore, decided to do something rather extraordinary and risky by literally removing the right hemisphere of Jodie's brain. This procedure is known as a 'hemispherectomy' and although risky, the results for Jodie were miraculous.

Along with her parents, the neurosurgeons were unsure of what to expect but were surprised and ecstatic to see her seizures end and a positive overall recovery. There were some minor post-operative challenges but with the help of physiotherapy Jodie not only survived but thrived. Although Jodie has limited movement in her left arm and a slight limp, she has grown into adulthood, graduated from college, received many scholarships and awards and is living a 'normal' and successful life, albeit with only half a brain. You see, at that young age Jodie's plastic brain reorganised itself and the left hemisphere took on the roles vacated by its counterpart. And while many other children suffering from Rasmussen's encephalitis have undergone successful hemispherectomies with equally miraculous outcomes, there is an important thing to remember … age makes a difference!

It is one thing to remove a major section of the brain in a young child but the outcome would be very different if performed on an adult. As we get older there is a degree of permanence that overshadows any substantive changes to the brain be they medical or through trauma or injury. Like wet cement, over time cement will harden and lose its malleability or 'plasticity'. So timing is everything and it is highly unlikely that removing half of your brain would end well. Relatedly, a young brain is far more susceptible to the environment. Children are indeed malleable, and when puberty kicks in the brain undergoes some substantive alterations and is vulnerable to whatever the environment has to offer. The next chapter helps us to understand how and why this occurs.

Summary

This chapter explored the remarkable complexity and plasticity of the human brain, describing how it develops from birth through adulthood. The brain contains trillions of neural connections—with one cubic millimetre storing approximately two thousand terabytes of data—and forms these connections through environmental experiences. The chapter examined key brain structures (brain stem, limbic system, and cerebrum) and their functions, highlighting the frontal lobes as the "CEO" of the brain which don't fully mature until around age 25. Two critical developmental processes were explained: "experience-expectant" stimulation (universal processes like vision development) and "experience-dependent" stimulation (individualised learning shaped by environment). The chapter also documented aspects of the brain's neuroplasticity—its ability to reorganise itself—which is particularly powerful during childhood and adolescence but diminishes with age. This understanding of brain development provides crucial context for understanding how environmental factors, including screen use, can shape neural pathways and behaviours during formative years.

Bibliography and Further Reading

Carter, R. (2009). *The Human Brain Book: An Illustrated Guide To Its Structure, Function and Disorders.* D.K. Publishing.

D'angelo, E. (2019). The cerebellum gets social. *Science*, 363(6424), 229. https://doi.org/10.1126/science.aaw2571.

Eagleman, D. (2020). *Livewired: The Inside Story of the Ever-Changing Brain.* Pantheon Books, New York.

Goldberg, E. (2001). *The Executive Brain: Frontal Lobes and the Civilized Mind.* Oxford University Press, Oxford, UK.

Hubel, D.H. & Wiesel, T.N. (1970). The period of susceptibility to the physiological effects of unilateral eye closure in kittens. *Journal of Physiology*, 206, 419–436.

LeDoux, J. (1998). *The Emotional Brain: The Mysterious Underpinnings of Emotional Life.* Simon & Schuster Inc, New York.

Mitchell, K. J. (2018). *Innate: How the Wiring of Our Brains Shapes Who We Are.* Princeton University Press.

Nagel, M. C. (2012). *In The Beginning: The Brain, Early Development and Learning.* Australian Council for Educational Research (ACER).

Nagel, M. C., & Scholes, L. (2016). Understanding Development and Learning: Implications for Teaching. Oxford University Press.

Pinker, S. (2009). *How the Mind Works.* W.W. Norton & Company.

Sweeney, M. S. (2009). *Brain, The Complete Guide: How It Develops, How It Works and How To Keep It Sharp.* National Geographic Society, Washington, D.C.

Voss, P., Thomas, M. E., Cisneros-Franco, J. M. & de Villers-Sidani, E. (2017). Dynamic brains and the changing rules of neuroplasticity: Implications for learning and recovery. *Frontiers in Psychology*, 8:1657.

2

Dude, Where's My Frontal Lobe?

We all meander out of childhood and into adult life through an adolescent door. Some adolescents go through it relatively easy, but most stumble over the threshold—their erratic (and alas often erotic) stumbling almost being a rite of passage.
—Robert Sylwester (2007, p. 1)

Abstract This chapter examines the neurodevelopmental changes that define adolescence, challenging the notion that teenage behaviour stems purely from hormonal changes. It frames the adolescent brain as undergoing significant reconstruction, with maturation progressing from the "reptile brain" (brainstem) and "monkey brain" (limbic system) to the "evolved brain" (cerebrum). Critically, while the limbic structures governing emotion, reward, and risk-taking—including the nucleus accumbens and amygdala—develop early, the prefrontal cortex responsible for impulse control, decision-making, and empathy lags behind, not fully maturing until the mid-twenties. This developmental mismatch explains many characteristic adolescent behaviours: impulsivity, emotional intensity, reward-seeking and poor risk assessment. The chapter highlights how synaptic pruning ("use it or lose it") and myelination shape neural

M. C. Nagel, R. Sharman, *Virtual Autism and Other Screen Disorders*, Palgrave Studies in Cyberpsychology, https://doi.org/10.1007/978-3-032-00803-9_2

pathways during this period, with environmental experiences playing a crucial role. The chapter also illuminates concerns related to how today's screen-dominated environment may negatively impact this critical developmental window, potentially interfering with healthy brain maturation in ways previous generations never experienced.

Keywords Adolescence • Pubescence • Frontal lobes • Theory of Mind • Myelin • Synaptic pruning • Amygdala • Nucleus accumbens

Remember When?!

Adolescence, or what some might call the teenage years ... do you remember that time? Can you recall things you might have said or done that drove the adults around you crazy? Did you saunter through the adolescent door into adulthood, or did you stumble, or did you often trip and fall? As we were putting this book together we shared some of our own adolescent escapades and were quickly reminded that in spite of all we have become, we were once the very beings many adults spend hours critiquing. We also remember that on more than one occasion we were asked, *why on God's green earth would you do that*, or something to that effect. In our discussions, Michael thought it apropos to share a story to remind everyone that while adults expend a great deal of energy lamenting today's youth, they too likely spent time stumbling through the door towards adulthood when puberty kicked in. To help the narrative, Michael will tell his story firsthand.

I grew up in the province of Saskatchewan in Canada's agricultural heartland. My mother and father were certainly 'old school'. Mum grew up in a Ukrainian community and didn't learn to speak English until she entered the formal years of schooling. She also left home at a very young age due to being the youngest of nine whose mother struggled to care for after her father passed away from complications arising from polio. Traditional Eastern European values shaped her worldview and work ethic which meant that while raising her three children she also worked as a short-order cook to help make ends meet.

My father was a mountain of a man, his German lineage evident in the large shadow his frame cast in the sunlight. He stood six foot two or 1.88 metres with broad shoulders, powerful arms, hands and visible strength that served him well as a blue-collar steel worker. Like many previous generations of parents, mine worked very hard, and at the same place, for most of their adult lives. They also worked hard at home and were committed to ensuring that my brother, sister and I were respectful of our 'elders' and teachers, disciplined, and applied ourselves at school to achieve and get the most out of life. And now the recollection. By some estimations, especially my sister's, my life was nearly cut short during the course of this event when my 14-year-old brain ensured that I stumbled, no, tripped through the adolescent door.

One day as my family was beginning to gather around the dinner table for the evening meal the telephone rang and like Pavlov's dog, my sister and I instantly reacted, not by salivating, but by hurling ourselves towards the phone on the wall near the table. We needed to answer in case it was a friend or in the event we could use the person on the other end to embarrass one another. My sister often took great delight in announcing that the person on the other end of the line was looking to speak to me and was a 'giirrrlll'. It's important to bear in mind that this was a time today's adolescents cannot relate to, a time when the phone was something not transportable. The ringing of the phone as it reverberated off the wall was my generation's equivalent of a notification alerting me to my own self-importance and need to get to the phone first, which I did.

At the same time my sister and I were racing to the phone, my dad had just arrived home from a 12-hour shift at the steel mill. His face was weary and although he washed his hands, the remnants of his day overshadowed his clothing and gruff demeanour. He looked tired and when in this state my dad was not open to conversation or doing anything other than eating and resting his body on the sofa. None of that mattered really because I was having a great time talking on the phone and making faces at my sister. Now here is where things get interesting.

Can you recall a moment in your life when time seemed to stand still? On this day in my life the universe stopped for me. At that moment, with my own perfect timing only a few moments after answering the phone, my dad went to sit down and I engaged in a school boy prank by pulling the chair out from under him. Time started to waver while I watched, in slow motion, my dad violently hitting the floor hard and my life flash before my eyes.

Did I mention my dad had big hands and my parents were old school? Now pulling the chair out from a classmate is one thing but doing so to your six foot two, two-hundred-and-twenty-pound mountain of a steel-worker father is something completely different. My mum stood there in shock. My brother, who is six years younger than me, stared in dumb-founded disbelief and my 12-year-old sister's face exuded an inner delight knowing what was likely to come next.

As my dad rose to his feet the steel mill induced weariness in his eyes evaporated and was replaced with the purest version of rage I had ever seen. This contrasted sharply with my mother's face showing the inner workings of her mind as she tried to work out how to navigate the storm ahead and protect her eldest cub. For me, I could feel the blood rush from my face as I solemnly bid my friend a fond adieu not knowing if I would ever see or speak to him again. Anxiety and fear caused my body to tighten but fight or flight was not an option. As he composed himself and stood up, my dad's icy stare penetrated my brain, and he bellowed out 'why on earth would you do that' (profanities omitted in the interests of good taste). I, in turn, answered with a gulp of air, and a genuine sense of bewilderment, 'I don't know'. Needless to say, the fact that you are reading about my story shows that I survived that lapse of judgement, barely!

Due to our own personal experiences as adolescents and more recently as the parents of adolescents we would contend most readers of the story above have had experience either asking and/or being asked a version of *why would you do that*. We would also argue that most adults conveniently or selectively forgot their adolescent moments as they bemoan or decry today's youth. Relatedly, it is unlikely any parent willingly shares their own adolescent indiscretions with their own children keeping such secrets buried for as long as humanly possible. Adult memories become selective or blurred when one moves through the adolescent door into adulthood.

Now a consideration related to stories of adolescent mayhem and poor decisions is what is it that can compel an adolescent to do things that might make their much younger siblings cringe in disbelief? Part of that answer can be found in brain. You see, it turns out there are many changes going on inside the brains of adolescents. We would argue that those changes, which are not visible, are unmatched by the physical changes that accompany puberty as sex hormones start doing the job of transitioning the body of a child into that of an adult.

Hormonal changes and associated physiological and physical changes in adolescence have been studied for years. At the turn of the twentieth century, G. Stanley Hall, considered one of psychology's founding fathers, described adolescence as a "period of storm and stress".[1] Even Aristotle held certain views on this stage of life and suggested that youth "are heated by nature as drunken men by wine".[2] Over time and across generations, advances in neuroscience and technology have informed us that periods of storms and stress and the heating of youth goes well beyond hormones. There are some significant and amazing developmental changes to the adolescent brain that play a part in understanding how adolescents think, or perhaps don't, and how they experience emotions and by association how they behave.

The Adolescent Brain

Before we look at the myriad of changes that occur in the brain during adolescence some clarity in definitions and terms is warranted. First, while some might like to use the phrase 'teen brain' when looking at brain maturation, we avoid doing so because too often this suggests a definitive timeline from 13 to 19; the brain is changing before and after those chronological bookends.

While we use the term adolescence with reference to brain maturation, we link it to the word pubescence. Adolescence can be vague given different social and cultural views about what adolescence might be which is where pubescence is helpful. Pubescence is a medical term denoting developmental changes to the reproductive system of a person and it is

[1] Hall (1904), Volume 1, p. xiii.

[2] Arnett (1999, p. 317).

significant to keep in mind that puberty does not start at 13! Some girls, for example, experience their first menarche (period) at age 10 with the average age of onset being 12.4 years.[3] Relatedly, puberty is also the time when we start to see developmental changes in the brain. Therefore, we us the term adolescence as a period recognising developmental changes to the body and brain from roughly 10 years to 20 years of age. In fact, full maturation of the brain is not complete until the mid-twenties but most of the hard work is done in the time frame we have identified. To simplify things we use the term 'adolescent brain' to acknowledge that most of the substantive changes to one's brain as a result of maturation occur somewhere between 10 and 20 years of age with some fine-tuning afterwards.

Second, while adolescence can indeed be a time of storm and stress, many adolescents navigate this storm with minimal difficulties so it's best not to over-generalise. We should not assume all adolescents are the same or are deficient due to the changes that are occurring. Yes, some will display greater anxiety or stress than others, which can impact on their well-being, relationships, education and future. Many more will get along well with others most of the time, succeed in school and life, become healthy productive adults and not fall into a pit of delinquency.[4]

Finally, it is important to emphasise that the adolescent brain is under massive reconstruction and is a work in progress. The remodelling of some of its basic structures coupled with fluctuations of hormones and neurotransmitters can impact on everything from eating and sleeping, to logic and language to impulses and intuition. So substantive are changes to the brain during adolescence that they have provided enough material for whole volumes of work on the topic, which go beyond what we need to do here. Instead, we will focus on some of the most significant changes that, in turn, might help you understand why your happy eight-year-old may have morphed into an emotionally charged, sensation-seeking creature who often resembles a character from apocalyptic zombie movie due to sleep deprivation and task avoidance disorder (not a medically recognised diagnosable disorder, just our way of remembering our own

[3] Marques et al. (2022).

[4] Nagel (2014); see also Arnett (1999); Masten et al. (1999, 2012); Dahl (2004); Steinberg et al. (2006).

children). Focusing on these changes also provides a framework for our contention that screen devices and their associated apps are having a net overall effect on young people. To that end, the best place to start is to revisit some of the information covered in the previous chapter and then look at the brain's CEO!

Three Brains in One

The first chapter offered some insights into major regions of the brain including the brain stem, limbic system, cerebellum and cerebrum. Using the work of Dr Paul D MacLean, we would like to extend that material to connect your thoughts to adolescents in a more primal way.

Dr Paul MacLean was a pioneering physician and neuroscientist who made substantive contributions across many disciplines including psychiatry, physiology and neuroscience. Most of his work was done at Yale Medical School and the National Institute of Mental Health in the United States. In the 1960s, MacLean suggested that the human brain was actually three brains in one when he proposed his evolutionary theory as a model referred to as the 'triune' brain.[5] He referred to these three brains as the reptilian complex, the paleomammalian complex and the neomammalian complex and viewed each as independently conscious entities that basically evolved from the bottom up. While the reptilian brain in MacLean's model focused mostly on the basal ganglia we could insert brainstem here, with the paleomammalian brain encompassing the limbic system and the neomammalian brain being that of the cerebrum. MacLean's model, which has not gone uncontested by other scientists, does give us an opportunity to poke a bit of fun at adolescents (a natural adult tendency) and rebadge things to help us remember what happens in each of these regions. So, let's call these regions the reptile brain (brainstem), the monkey brain (limbic system) and the evolved brain (cerebrum).

The reptile brain initiates and maintains many activities that can be primal, often reactionary and without filters. These can include

[5] MacLean's model was developed in the 1960s and later published as a volume of work in 1990 (see bibliography for full reference).

breathing, sweating, shivering, pooing, weeing, farting, burping, thirst, hunger, fighting, fleeing, freezing and sex. The monkey brain adds another layer to those primal urges by overlapping each with a range of emotions; being sad, angry, happy, disgusted, ashamed and so on. The evolved brain is another layer of sophistication that can curtail or shall we say corral the reptile and monkey brain by putting the brakes on unabashed impulses or emotional overload. For adolescents however, those brakes are faulty leaving them to the whims of their reptile and monkey motivations. Adolescents often want, and act, like lizard monkeys. Much of their time is spent seeking new and novel experiences and sensations, striving for independence, and experimenting and testing boundaries often without thinking through their actions or responsibilities. All these things are part of an adolescent's journey towards shaping their identity (covered in detail in Chap. 7). However, some important maturational changes in the brain means an adolescent will often act without thinking; the lizard monkey is stepping on the gas while the brakes need refurbishing.

A good beginning to better understand why adolescents can present some challenging and puzzling behaviours is to cut to the chase and focus on the part of the brain that will, eventually, be better able to curb the lizard monkey. That part of the brain includes the frontal lobes and in particular, the right prefrontal cortex. The previous chapter offered some important foundational information about the frontal lobes but greater detail is required here.

Our frontal lobes are what separate us from all other species and places humans at the top of the proverbial food chain. Lizards and monkeys can do many things but their brains pale in comparison to what our frontal lobes allow us to do. Our frontal lobes not only play an active role in monitoring and regulating most everything our lizard and monkey brains would like to do, but they are also the epicentre of our minds. Decision-making, responsible thinking, planning, anticipation, attention, concentration, analysis, empathy, sequencing, learning from errors and various other higher-order thinking skills all reside in, or are a part of, the brain's frontal lobes. Damage to this region of the brain can lead to untold consequences and influence everything from temperament to judgement to personality to, well you're getting the picture, most everything that makes us human. The story of Phineas Gage offers real-life evidence to this claim.

In 1848, Phineas Gage, a 25-year-old railroad construction worker survived a very harrowing experience. On September 13, Gage was part of a group blasting rock to make way for railroad lines. He was assigned to placing gunpowder in a deep hole and while pressing the gunpowder into the hole with an iron crowbar, sparks ignited the gunpowder resulting in that iron bar perforating Gage's skull. The bar entered his left cheek, destroying his eye while passing through the front left of the brain and exiting the skull. The bar itself was 3.2 centimetres in diameter and basically created a channel through Gage's head.[6]

That Phineas Gage even survived his ordeal is a miracle given the initial loss of blood, the fact that the wound became badly infected and the state of medical care at this time in history. His physical condition slowly improved however what was more astonishing than him surviving was what happened to his persona. Prior to the accident, and by most accounts, Gage appeared a well-mannered, affable man and was considered the most capable employee of the company who demonstrated a well-balanced mind and sense of leadership.[7] After the accident, his once gentle personality began to decline. He became bad mannered and disrespectful to his colleagues, irritable, irreverent, rude and prone to swearing. Gage was essentially no longer himself nor someone that his friends and acquaintances wanted to spend any time with or be in his company.[8] The tragedy of Phineas Gage demonstrated to doctors and researchers the important range of functions of the frontal lobes. We now know that damage to the prefrontal lobes, especially during childhood, can not only impair many important functions related to thinking and consciousness but also demonstrably change one's personality.[9]

By now it should be self-evident that our frontal lobes play perhaps the most critical role in defining who we are and what we do and are the last regions of the brain to fully mature. For adolescents this has many implications. Consider, for example, the potential challenges when the mechanisms for mediating and helping to channel and harness the seething

[6] MacMillan (2002).

[7] Teles (2020).

[8] Ibid. See also, Barker (1995).

[9] Bahia et al. (2013).

energy of emotions within the limbic system are not fully developed. Aside from helping to regulate emotions, it is the prefrontal lobes that guide other parts of the brain including the regions that govern motivation, decision-making and rewards. Immature prefrontal lobes in adolescents result in them being hotwired for emotional, risky, sensation-seeking behaviour but too often unable to think through the consequences of their actions.

It is interesting to note that brain imaging has shown that an adolescent brain literally looks different from that of both a child and adult.[10] The fact that the immature adolescent frontal lobes do not appear 'adult-like' is arguably observable in many of the challenges and debates concerning adolescent behaviour including drug use, risk-taking, sexual behaviour and screen time. Neuroscientist and author, Professor Frances E Jensen suggests that the adolescent brain is not just an adult brain with fewer miles on it, it is in essence a different kind of brain altogether.[11]

While many might agree from anecdotal experience that the adolescent brain is 'a different brain altogether', this is not a license to excuse adolescents for less than desirable behaviour. Rather, it is important to keep in mind that the frontal lobes are in a state of transformation, that this will take some time and as such adolescent behaviour and decision-making can be problematic. Couple this with the truism that consistently making good decisions is not always a reasonable expectation of a mature adult brain and we might be more willing to accord some measure of understanding and empathy when adolescents make a bad choice.

So with this knowledge in mind, why did Michael tempt fate by pulling the chair out from his father? Why could he not articulate a motivation? Without those frontal lobes, the ability to hypothesise, forecast forward, weigh options and hit the brakes on an initiated action is severely diminished. Alternatively, the lizard-monkey brain is a stimulus response machine. See a glass of water (stimulus), you drink it (response). But what if it's not your water? What if it's contaminated? Those questions are asked by the frontal lobe, and as you reach for the cup, you do a double

[10] Wilbrecht (2018); for insights into differences evident through scanning see Giedd et al. (1996); Giedd (2004); Durston et al. (2006).

[11] As discussed in Bryson (2019). For a full copy of Professor Jensen's commentary see Ruder (2008).

take and retract your hand. Add a few years and you won't even initiate that action in the first place as your frontal lobes increase in speed of processing and analysis and pre-empt the lizard monkey's ill thought through response.

Michael's lizard brain saw the chair and his father attempting to sit, his monkey brain remembered a prank and how funny it is. Action was initiated. Quite literally without thought to the difference in circumstances and likely outcome. No brakes were invoked. Only after the outcome became immediately apparent did a double take (and rethink) occur. This is classic teenage brain behaviour, and Michael was genuine in his motivation when he exclaimed 'I don't know'.

This is in fact, the basis of the well-known Hanlon's razor:

Never attribute to malice that which is adequately explained by stupidity.

Malice requires a surprising amount of frontal lobe activity: memory, attribution and suppression of immediate reaction (impulse) vs planning a more strategic revenge (a dish served cold). Stupidity on the other hand relies on the lizard-monkey system with frontal lobes in absentia. If people tell you they honestly don't know why they did something incredibly stupid, they're probably telling you the truth.

I Know What You're Thinking!

Imagine this … it's late in the afternoon and while you are sitting in your kitchen, out of the corner of your eye you see a family member open the refrigerator and start perusing its shelves. It is likely that the first thing that comes to your mind is that that person is hungry and so you interrupt what you're doing and let them know that there are some leftovers on the bottom shelf or that there are biscuits in the pantry. In that brief moment what you have done is exercise a basic aspect of Theory of Mind (ToM).

ToM is the ability to think about what another person is thinking or more simply stated, the ability to put yourself in another person's shoes. This is an aspect of what we call social cognition. It not only includes the ability to understand and predict another person's mental processes including their emotions, thoughts, intentions, beliefs and motives but also permits us to think about our own mental state.[12] Our ability to figuratively read someone else's mind gives us a crucial evolutionary advantage over all other species in that it allows us to better interact with the environment and cooperate more efficiently with others.[13] Being able to predict the feelings of another human being is critical to connecting with others and forming relationships. Consider also that observed deficits in ToM are part of a broad range of symptoms in schizophrenia, bipolar disorder, some forms of dementia, 'psychopathy' and other psychiatric disorders. ToM also appears to be selectively impaired in autistic spectrum disorders leaving other cognitive functions intact.[14] Just to emphasise and to keep in mind when we discuss the potential impact of screen devices on the brain, ToM appears impaired in individuals with autistic spectrum disorder.

The chronology of the emergence of ToM as we mature is, to date, somewhat contentious. There is evidence to suggest that it does not appear to be present at birth, seems to emerge around four or five years of age and adolescents do not appear to have a ToM as fully developed as that of adults.[15] Indeed, adolescence is a crucial period in terms of the emergence and development of ToM.

To reiterate, ToM emerges over time and this chronology of development is directly linked to the frontal lobes. Indeed, to effectively think about your own mental state or the thoughts and feelings of others relies a great deal on activity in the frontal lobes. This also shows us that ToM is part of a sophisticated relationship between the brain's CEO and its emotional heart. In order to be socially effective, build relationships, regulate one's emotions while understanding a range of emotions in others requires control over, and a capacity for integrating, the full range of thinking and emotional processes.[16] For adolescents, such activities are

---

[12] Nagel (2012).

[13] Cuzzolin et al. (2020).

[14] Brüne and Brüne-Cohrs (2006).

[15] Nagel (2014); see also Blakemore (2008); Sebastian et al. (2012); Weimer et al. (2017).

[16] Meinhardt-Injac et al. (2020).

not easily done given that their brains are still maturing. Perspective-taking, reading social cues and other aspects of ToM take time and a range of experiences to ensure healthy development. Never forget, there is a great deal going on in the brains of adolescents, which, in turn, impacts on all aspects of the mind.

Their Changing Minds!

The description of the development and importance of ToM in association with the maturation of the frontal lobes is just one story of what is occurring in the minds of adolescents. There are others and they also impact on most aspects of thinking and behaviour. These stories are multi-layered and integrated with one another. They are worthy of some consideration, however, as they help to further clarify why an adolescent who might physically look like an adult, is simply a different creature altogether.

Let's start by looking back! If you recall from chapter one, the brain is comprised of an unimaginable labyrinth of neural connectivity. Synapses, or the passing of information from one neuron to the other is both the process and product of this connectivity. Right now your brain is busy sending trillions of bits and pieces of information from one region to the other. Your eyes are sending the text you are reading to your occipital lobes which in turn are using regions of the left temporal lobe to decipher the words on this page. The sensations in and around your body, most of which you are not consciously aware are being interpreted for any action necessary. If the ambient temperature of the room starts to increase, your brain may automatically start all the mechanics necessary for you to perspire to help you cool down or send you to get a cold drink of water. Again, so much is going on in your brain that you are not aware of thanks to the myriad of connections that ensure our survival and our capacity to engage with the world around us. And while those connections are integral to our existence, there is a material that ensures they work expediently and efficiently.

Have you heard of myelin? Perhaps not but maybe you have heard that the brain has grey and white matter. The white matter of the brain is actually myelin and without getting to technical myelin is a fatty material consisting of a number of materials including proteins and cholesterol. At birth we have very limited amounts of myelin but this fatty material will increase well into our twenties ... in essence we become fatheads as we mature. You may be asking yourself why all this chatter about fat in our heads. Well, turns out that the more myelin you have the better your brain works. You see, myelin wraps around parts of a neuron called the axon which in turn makes the passing of electrical impulses work faster and with greater efficiency. A good analogy is the plastic coating around copper wiring which protects the wiring thereby allowing electricity to flow freely. Take away that plastic coating leaving the wire exposed and you increase the likelihood of things going wrong. The same can be said about myelin. For example, the immune system attacks myelin and the cells that produce it in individuals with multiple sclerosis.

As noted above, the immature brain of an infant has limited amounts of myelin. Over time this important fatty material will increase and in conjunction with experiences from the surrounding environment will shape the neural superhighway of the brain. Myelin grows in fits and starts around different regions of the brain over time and increases about 100% during adolescence allowing neural messages to travel faster and with greater proficiency. Keep in mind that when talking about the passing of information from one neuron to another, we are talking milliseconds in spite of the extended blank gaze you may encounter when questioning an adolescent's motives or behaviour. Interestingly, while there is a build-up of myelin and a strengthening of neural connections during adolescence, there is also a state of deconstruction going on.

If you recall from the previous chapter, we noted that the brain of an infant has more neurons than it needs. By three years of age a child will have more neural connections than its paediatrician. In a sense the brain overcompensates its connectivity to ensure healthy neural development. During adolescence that same brain will begin a journey of eliminating many of those connections through a process known as synaptic 'pruning'.

Synaptic pruning is a very important aspect of neural refinement during adolescence. All of the connections formed in the early stages of life are simply not necessary. The brain, therefore, gets rid of those connections linked to actions, activities and experiences no longer practised or important and strengthens those connections that are repeatedly activated. In more colloquial terms researchers refer to this process as 'use it or lose it'.[17] To perhaps help you better understand this, Michael has another adolescent anecdote.

Je Ne Sais Pas!

Around the same time I was pulling a chair out from under my father I was in the midst of a grade seven educational dilemma, or at least that is what my adolescent brain thought at the time. In grade seven, or year seven as they say in Australia, students in Saskatchewan are introduced to something that is arguably of little interest to many, if not most adolescents. It's a subject called French.

Growing up in the prairies I knew there was a province called Quebec and that Canada had two official languages. I knew this because my favourite ice hockey team at the time was the Montreal Canadians and every bit of junk food I bought had the ingredients listed in two languages; such was my limited interest in a province hundreds of kilometres away. This all changed the first week of school when a teacher walked into our class with resources I could not read and started speaking to us in a language I could not, and did not, want to know. The language was French. This subject and classroom practice continued in eighth grade and over time I did manage to learn how to utter various shades of what I now consider a beautiful language. However, the only part of French that still resides in my now aged brain is one phrase in particular, *je ne sais pas*—translation, *I don't know*! Je ne sais pas was the term I used the most and all other aspects of French I learned were lost. Eighth grade was the last year of compulsory French and my adolescent brain busily discarded unused language connections, what I used the most stayed and all else disappeared.

[17] Shamay-Tsoory et al. (2010).

The example above arguably oversimplifies the intricacies of synaptic pruning but does offer some sense of what happens when the adolescent brain is busy refining itself. Something worth remembering, however, is the role of the environment in shaping the connections of an adolescent's brain. In a Shakespearean sense, to use it or lose it, is to be or not to be. To be doing things repeatedly has an impact on the brain and overall development and since the turn of the century, adolescent 'being' has increasingly witnessed time spent on screens, and existing forever elsewhere. Some have gone so far as to refer to adolescents as 'screenagers' given the time spent immersed in devices and in particular smartphones. Worryingly, debates around whether time on screens is impacting the brains of young people no longer can be answered with je nais se pas. We do know the answer to that question and are only beginning to understand the deleterious outcomes of spending too much time in a virtual world but we will leave that for later chapters.

Controlling the Lizard Monkey

Okay, so now that you know the importance of myelin and using it or losing it there is one last discussion necessary in helping to understand the developing adolescent brain. This discussion starts in noting that with all that is going on inside the heads of adolescents, the brain matures roughly from the bottom (lizard brain) up to the top (cerebrum), around to the front and from the inside (monkey brain) out. This maturational journey occurs at a different rate for males and females and females are generally a couple of years ahead of males in most aspects of development. This is important because regions of the lizard-monkey brain associated with survival, emotions and rewards mature sooner than the higher-order thinking areas of the frontal lobes. Two structures in the lizard-monkey brain that likely influence behaviour are the nucleus accumbens and amygdala (Fig. 2.1).

Although debatable, there is ample evidence, both scientific and anecdotal, to suggest that perhaps the most primal driver of human behaviour is pleasure seeking associated with rewards. This is likely a truism of all living creatures as it appears that every living thing is willing to expend a

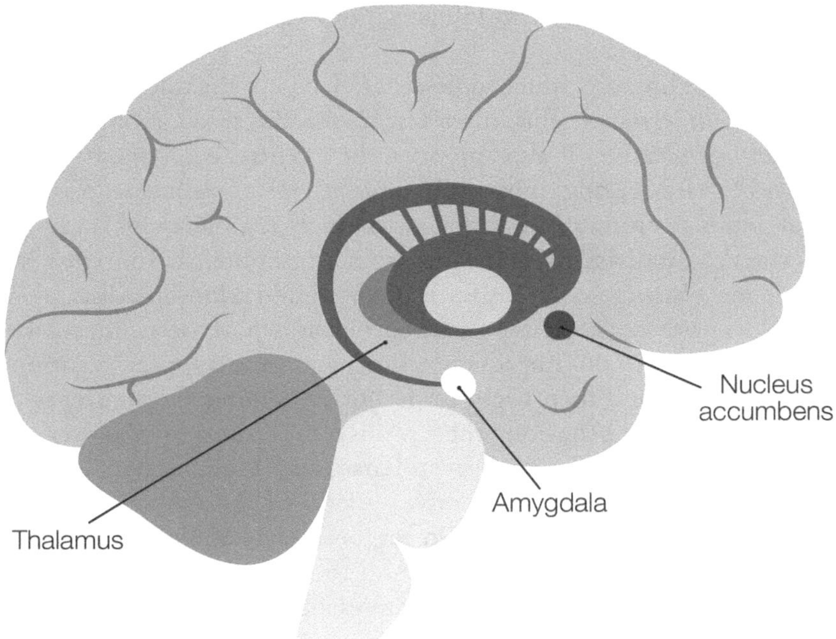

Fig. 2.1 Amygdala and nucleus accumbens in limbic system

certain amount of effort in order to seek something desirable or some sort of reward. Behavioural psychologists and researchers have identified such behaviours in animals and human beings and noted regions of the brain that play a role in such activity.[18] In humans, the nucleus accumbens is worthy of consideration.[19]

The nucleus accumbens is a central part of the limbic system that resides deep in the brain. It is activated during pleasant or emotionally arousing experiences and is a key player in the reward circuitry of the brain. A functioning nucleus accumbens relies on a couple of neurotransmitters, most notably dopamine, the chemical that promotes desire and

[18] Nagel (2014).

[19] The seminal works of BF Skinner can be found in any psychology text. His research and development of the theory of Operant Conditioning is evident in how parents and teachers reward and punish children to sustain or change behaviour. For insights into the reward systems and emotions in human and non-human species see Nagel (2014, 2019); Panksepp (2004, 2014).

pleasure and serotonin which influences our sense of satiety, inhibition, calmness and wellbeing.

In terms of understanding adolescent behaviour, the role of dopamine cannot be understated. This important chemical is much more than just a marker for pleasure. It also appears to be a central component in novelty and reward-seeking, motivation and feelings of wellbeing. So influential is this neurotransmitter that exceedingly high levels of dopamine are evident in individuals who suffer from schizophrenia, Tourette's syndrome and obsessive-compulsive disorder while Parkinson's disease and difficulties with maintaining attention on tasks have been linked with low levels. Levels of this important neurochemical also appear to rise during adolescence and then begin to decline as adulthood approaches. In terms of adolescent behaviour, there seems to be a 'dopamine' power-play between the higher order, and yet still maturing, thinking regions of the brain, and the more primal emotive systems of the monkey brain. In practical terms this often results in responsible decision-making giving way to impulsivity and risk-taking. And to make adolescent behaviour even more interesting, risk taking promotes increases in dopamine, which may predispose adolescents to further risk-taking; a circuitous biochemical circuit that likely gets many adolescents into trouble. This is not to suggest that all adolescents will indulge in varying degrees of risky behaviour, but many certainly do.

Of further interest in the discussion is that during adolescence and most predominantly in the teenage years, receptors in the nucleus accumbens are engorged with dopamine but because the brain is still maturing there is often a disconnect between the effort expended and the desire for a reward. In the day-today reality of adolescence, this means that young people tend to prefer activities that require relatively low to moderate effort yet produce immediate high rewards. Adolescents will look for a quick dopamine hit without having to do much thinking about it. Sensation-seeking and risk-taking behaviours ranging from playing video games to skateboarding to riding on the tops of trains to sexual behaviours to experimenting with alcohol and drugs can become part of that dopamine rush. Sensation-seeking and risk-taking behaviours are important evolutionary drivers for becoming independent so should not be considered as wholly negative; taking risks is part of growing up, but doing so in a way that is prosocial, does not result in injuring or humiliating one's father at the dinner table and not a threat to life and limb is desirable.

Aside from the powerful impact resulting from the interplay of dopamine in the nucleus accumbens, the need for novelty and excitement through sensation seeking may also be influenced by the amygdala. Latin for almond due to its shape, the amygdala is a tiny structure that is also part of the limbic system and impact behaviour. There are actually two amygdalae residing in the temporal lobes but the two are generally considered one structure. The amygdala is a major processing centre for emotions and links emotions to other important activities including memory, learning and our senses. It is the amygdala that helps us respond emotionally to a range of experiences and most importantly it is part of our fight-or-flight response system. If you were walking past someone's yard and a barking dog lunged at the fence and startled you, your amygdala helps you to decide whether to stand your ground or make for the hills!

Standing your ground or running away is important albeit small roles that stem from the amygdala. The amygdala also plays a part in aggressive behaviour, learning through rewards and punishment, reading intentions of others, addiction and as noted earlier, memory. Remember too that the limbic system (monkey brain) matures sooner than the brain's CEO which is why adolescents can appear quite moody and misread emotional responses; they are more likely to overreact to any type of negative situation instead of reacting with the type of controlled response we might see in adults. In simpler terms, the amygdala is responsible for automatic 'hot' responses rather than 'cool' considered responses.

Another important feature that can emerge from an unchecked and mature amygdala is evident in the propensity for adolescents to misread neutral or inquisitive facial expressions as a sign of anger. In its entirety, it is the amygdala that can lead adolescents to feel that they live in a hostile and dangerous world and their hot response to this world may include various degrees of emotional overreaction and/or aggression ranging from rumour mongering in females to fisticuffs in males.

At this stage it should be evident that structural changes at the nexus of chemical and hormonal changes in the brain during adolescence are predictive of certain behaviours. These developmental inevitabilities are partially responsible for changing a child into a restless, exuberant and emotionally intense adolescent desperate to achieve every goal, experience every sensation and fulfil every desire where many feelings and perceptions are amplified and often unchecked. However, while these changes mark an important transition from child to adult as they help to build independence and identity, they can also lead to questionable decisions and a multitude of challenges beyond behavioural indiscretions.

An important caveat in the discussion above, however, is that regardless of the potential reckless nature of adolescents leading adults to think that young people underestimate risks when making decisions, it turns out that that may not necessarily be true. Instead, when making decisions, adolescents tend to overestimate rewards or rather, find rewards more rewarding than any risks associated with attaining those rewards. 'I'll take the carrot and worry about any stick later' is far more prevalent in adolescents as compared to adults. As noted earlier, this could be because the nucleus accumbens is much more active in adolescents as compared to children or adults. We contend also that this offers some understanding into why an adolescent's first love, sporting achievement or other novel experiences can bring on great emotional intensity. Moreover, such intensity can be amplified in many ways beyond athletics and friends, including the use of screen devices, which are designed to hook the user by elevating dopamine. This is something to be explored in the next couple of chapters but for now it should be abundantly clear that the adolescent brain is a work in progress.

The information above is but a snapshot of all the things going on in the developing adolescent brain. Only a snapshot indeed, but one that projects some of the important considerations related to the types of experiences young people are engaging in. Previous generations have always known that there are enormous challenges associated with raising and guiding such young minds into adulthood. We now believe that those past challenges have intensified through the interplay of a twenty-first century, 24/7 media rich world and a brain that took thousands of years to evolve. It is also interesting that while older generations have often bemoaned the plight of the current crop of adolescents, we also believe that today's young people actually face cultural and social changes impacting on their neural development in ways previous generations never experienced or were exposed to. This is exacerbated in the reality that today's young people take fewer opportunities to 'do' the types of activities that previous generations experienced and instead spend a great deal of time in a virtual world.

Finally, and before moving through the remaining chapters, it is important to remember that nature and nurture work in tandem to shape the brain. For example, as the prefrontal lobes of an adolescent mature, they get better at controlling impulses and thinking of others. However, such improvements also require cascades of interactions between individuals and the environment and multitudes of experiences that are intimately linked with 'learning'. We learn to make better decisions by making not-so-good decisions and then correcting our behaviour. We become better planners by making plans, implementing them and evaluating the results, again and again. Our social and cultural life is shaped by our biology and vice versa and as such dealing with today's adolescents is not as hopeless as the 'what could they be thinking' catchcry might suggest. It isn't that the adolescent brain's prefrontal lobes just don't show up when they need to, it's just that they need instruction and exercise. Crucially, such instruction and experience is more powerful and effective when it happens in a real world rather than a virtual one. In fact, there is much to suggest that the virtual world and too much time on screen are defective rather than effective in shaping the minds of young people. The rest of this book looks to expand on that claim, to provide evidence to support it and then outline strategies and ideas for counteracting it.

Summary

Chapter 2 examined the neurodevelopmental changes that define adolescence, challenging the notion that teenage behaviour stems purely from hormonal changes. It framed the adolescent brain as undergoing significant reconstruction, with maturation progressing from the "reptile brain" (brainstem) and "monkey brain" (limbic system) to the "evolved brain" (cerebrum). Critically, while the limbic structures governing emotion, reward, and risk-taking—including the nucleus accumbens and amygdala—develop early, the prefrontal cortex responsible for impulse control, decision-making, and empathy lags behind, not fully maturing until the mid-twenties. This developmental mismatch explains many characteristic adolescent behaviours: impulsivity, emotional intensity, reward-seeking and poor risk assessment. The chapter highlighted how synaptic pruning ("use it or lose it") and myelination shape neural pathways during this period, with environmental experiences playing a crucial role. The chapter also illuminated concerns related to how today's screen-dominated environment may negatively impact this critical developmental window, potentially interfering with healthy brain maturation in ways previous generations never experienced.

Bibliography and Further Reading

Arnett, J.J. (1999). Adolescent storm and stress, reconsidered. *American Psychologist*, 54(5), 317–326. https://doi.org/10.1037/0003-066X.54.5.317

Bahia, V.S., Takada, L.T., Caixeta, L., Lucato, L.T., Porto, C.S. & Nitrini, R. (2013). Prefrontal damage in childhood and changes in the development of personality: A case report. *Dementia Neuropsychologia*, 7(1), 132–135. https://doi.org/10.1590/S1980-57642013DN70100019

Barker, F.G. (1995). Phineas among the phrenologists: The American crowbar case and nineteenth-century theories of cerebral localization. *Journal of Neurosurgery*, 82(4), 672–682. https://doi.org/10.3171/jns.1995.82.4.0672

Blakemore, S.J. (2008). The social brain in adolescence. *Nature Reviews Neuroscience*, 9(4), 267–277. https://doi.org/10.1038/nm2353/

Brüne, M. & Brüne-Cohrs, U. (2006). Theory of mind – evolution, ontogeny, brain mechanisms and psychopathology. *Neuroscience and Biobehavioral Reviews*, 30(4), 437–455. https://doi.org/10.1016/j.neubiorev.2005.08.001.

Bryson, B. (2019). *The Body: The Guide for Occupants*. Doubleday.

Cuzzolin, F., Morelli, A., Cîrstea, B. & Sahakian, B.J. (2020). Knowing me, Knowing you: Theory of Mind in AI. *Psychological Medicine*, 50, 1057–1061. https://doi.org/10.1017/S0033291720000835.

Dahl, R.E. (2004). Adolescent brain development: A period of vulnerabilities or opportunities. *Annals of the New York Academy of Sciences*, 1021, 1–22. https://doi.org/10.1196/annals.1308.001

Durston, S., Davidson, M.C., Tottenham, N., Galvan, A., Spicer, J., Fossella, J.A. & Casey, B.J. (2006). A shift from diffuse to focal cortical activity with development. *Developmental Science*, 9(1), 1–8. https://doi.org/10.1111/j.1467-7687.2005.00454.x

Giedd, J.N. (2004). Structural magnetic resonance imaging of the adolescent brain. *Annals of the New York Academy of Sciences, 1021*(1), 77–85. https://doi.org/10.1196/annals.1308.009

Giedd, J.N., Vaituzis, C., Hamburger, S. D., Lange, N., Rajapakse, J. C., Kaysen, D., Vauss, Y. C., & Rapoport, J. L. (1996). Quantitative MRI of the temporal lobe, amygdala and hippocampus in normal human development: Ages 4–18 years. *Journal of Comparative Neurology, 366*(2), 223–230. https://doi.org/10.1002/(SICI)1096-9861(19960304)366:2<223::AID-CNE3>3.0.CO;2-7

Hall, G. (1904). *Adolescence: Its Psychology and Its Relations to Physiology, Anthropology, Sociology, Sex, Crime, Religion and Education (Volumes I & II)*. Prentice-Hall.

MacLean, P.D. (1990). *The Triune Brain in Evolution: Role in Paleocerebral Functions.* Springer.

MacMillan, M. (2002). *An Odd Kind of Fame. Stories of Phineas Gage*. MIT Press.

Marques, P. Madeira, T. & Gama, A. (2022). Menstrual cycle among adolescents: Girl's awareness and influence of age at menarche and overweight. *Revista Paulista de Pediatria*, Jan 5, 40:e2020494. https://doi.org/10.1590/1984-0462/2022/40/2020494

Masten, A.S., Hubbard, J.J., Gest, S.D., Tellegen, A., Garmezy, N. & Ramirez, M. (1999). Competence in the context of adversity: Pathways to resilience and maladaptation from childhood to late adolescence. *Development and Psychopathology*, 11 (1), 143–169. https://doi.org/10.1017/s0954579499001996

Masten, C.L., Telzer, E.H., Fuligni, A.J., Lieberman, M.D. & Eisenberger, N.I. (2012). Time spent with friends in adolescence relates to less neural sensitivity to later peer rejection. *Social Cognitive and Affective Neuroscience*, 7(1), 106–114. https://doi.org/10.1093/scan/nsq098

Meinhardt-Injac, B., Dau, M.M. & Meinhardt, G. (2020). Theory of mind development from adolescence to adulthood: Testing the two-component model. *British Journal of Developmental Psychology*, 38(2), 289–303. https://doi.org/10.1111/bjdp.12320.

Nagel, M. C. (2012). *In The Beginning: The Brain, Early Development and Learning*. Australian Council for Educational Research (ACER).

Nagel, M.C. (2014). *In the Middle: The Adolescent Brain, Behaviour and Learning*. Australian Council for Educational Research (ACER).

Nagel, M.C. (2019). Neurobiology of risk taking and impulsivity. In M. Nagel & R Sharman (Eds.), *The Encyclopedia of Child and Adolescent Development, Vol 8 – Biology, Neurology and Cognition in Adolescence* (pp. 1–8). Wiley-Blackwell Publishing Ltd. https://doi.org/10.1002/9781119171492.wecad361

Panksepp, J. (2004). *Affective Neuroscience: The Foundations of Human and Animal Emotions*. Oxford University Press.

Panksepp, J. (2014). Integrating bottom-up internalist views of emotional feelings with top-down externalist views: Might brain affective changes constitute reward and punishment effects within animal brains? *Cortex*, 59, 208–213. https://doi.org/10.1016/j.cortex.2014.04.15

Ruder, D. B. (2008). A work in progress: The teen brain. *Harvard Review*, 3(1), 8–10.

Sebastian, C.L., Fontaine, N.M.G., Bird, G., Blakemore, S.J., De Brito, S.A., McCrory, E.J.P. & Viding, E. (2012). Neural processing associated with cognitive and affective Theory of Mind in adolescents and adults. *Social Cognitive and Affective Neuroscience*, 7(1), 53–63. https://doi.org/10.1093/scan/nsr023.

Shamay-Tsoory, S.G., Harari, H., Aharon-Peretz, J. & Levkovitz, Y. (2010). The role of the orbitofrontal cortex in affective theory of mind deficits in criminal offenders with psychopathic tendencies. *Cortex*, 46(5), 668–677. https://doi.org/10.1016/j.cortex.2009.04.008.

Steinberg, L., Dahl, R., Keating, D., Kupfer, D.J., Masten, A.S. & Pine, D.S. (2006). The study of developmental psychopathology in adolescence: Integrating affective neuroscience with the study of context. In D Cicchetti & D.J. Cohen, (Eds.), *Developmental Psychopathology, Vol 2: Developmental Neuroscience,* 2nd Ed., (pp. 710–741). John Wiley & Sons Inc.

Teles, R.V. (2020). Phineas Gage's great Legacy. *Dementia & Neuropsychologia*, 14(4), 419–421. https://doi.org/10.1590/1980-57642020dn14-040013

Weimer, A.A., Parault Dowds, S.J., Fabricius, W.V., Schwanenflugel, P.J., & Suh, G.W. (2017). Development of constructivist theory of mind from middle childhood to early adulthood and its relation to social cognition and behavior. *Journal of Experimental Child Psychology, 154*, 28–45. https://doi.org/10.1016/j.jecp.2016.10.002.

Wilbrecht, L. (2018). Your twelve-year-old isn't just sprouting new hair but is also forming (and being formed by) new neural connections. In D. J. Linden (Ed.), *Think Tank: Forty Neuroscientists Explore the Roots of Human Experience* (pp. 45–51). Yale University Press.

3

Living in Our Matrix

This is your last chance. After this, there is no turning back. You take the blue pill—the story ends, you wake up in your bed and believe whatever you want to believe. You take the red pill—you stay in Wonderland and I show you how deep the rabbit hole goes.
—Morpheus, The Matrix

Abstract This chapter investigates how screen technology has fundamentally altered human reality, drawing parallels to the film "The Matrix" where humans navigate dual realities. It critically assesses many educational system's embrace of digital technologies, challenging the assumption that computers inherently improve learning outcomes. Evidence from OECD reports and research studies suggests minimal or negative correlations between heavy ICT investment and academic achievement. The chapter also explores three key concerns related to screen usage: increased sedentary behaviour among children, diminished cognitive performance from multi-tasking, and disruptions to sleep patterns and social development. Despite significant financial investment in classroom technology, research indicates these devices may contribute to poorer academic outcomes and compromised wellbeing. Questions around whether

M. C. Nagel, R. Sharman, *Virtual Autism and Other Screen Disorders*, Palgrave Studies in Cyberpsychology, https://doi.org/10.1007/978-3-032-00803-9_3

educational technology initiatives represent worthwhile investments or whether they inadvertently contribute to developmental issues in young people are also interrogated. In the end the research offered promotes the advocacy of a more balanced approach that views screen devices as occasional tools rather than educational necessities, enabling students to thrive in genuine human interactions rather than becoming immersed in a digital matrix.

Keywords Information and Computer Technologies (ICTs) • Organisation for Economic Co-operation and Development (OECD) • Programme for International Student Assessment (PISA) • Sedentary behaviour • Metabolic syndrome • Multi-tasking • Cognitive bottleneck • Working memory • Sleep

The Technological Rabbit Hole

Imagine living in two worlds, two realities! In 1999 the hit movie *The Matrix* posited that story to its millions of viewers by introducing us to the main character, Thomas Anderson, played by Keanu Reeves. Thomas is a computer programmer by day but at night he thrives as a computer hacker with the alias of *Neo*. Neo spends much of his time questioning reality. He is also consumed by repeated online encounters with the phrase 'The Matrix'. He senses that some sort of 'sign' will come his way and enlighten him about this 'Matrix'. Little does Neo know but his sense of reality is rapidly thrown on its head when he encounters another character, Morpheus, who offers him a blue or red pill. Neo takes the red pill and soon learns that The Matrix, is a computer-generated dream world of binary code designed by machines to keep humans under control. In the movie humans are kept sedated and are effectively living a virtual life. In his new reality, Neo discovers that what he considered to be the real world as a computer programmer is actually nothing more than a computer program created by a malevolent Artificial Intelligence. In fact, Neo finds that his reality is a façade for sentient machines who grow and harvest people to use as an ongoing energy source.

Once again, imagine living in two worlds, two realities. We think that yesterday's science fiction about a dystopian existence where machines monitor and dictate human reality is perhaps not too far removed from today's reality. Consider that one of the key messages in The Matrix and its two sequels focuses on notions of agency and freewill and could be applied today. Specifically, this message contends that everyone has the individual responsibility to make the choice between how much time they spend in the real world of human beings or in an artificial world to be found via technology. We would like to suggest that with each passing year since the release of The Matrix and the ubiquitous incursion of technology in our lives, that choice is becoming increasingly worthy of scrutiny as younger and younger children are spending more and more time in virtual worlds. It would also seem that making a choice to be in the real world is becoming increasingly difficult. Today's youth are consumed by a world of binary code as purposefully designed advanced algorithms curate their online interests and activities to keep them immersed in a digitised reality.

Now some of you may be thinking that human beings have meandered through a long history of technological advancements, and we would agree. However, perhaps no measure of advancement has been as pervasive and omnipotent as that afforded to us via binary code and screen devices. Such a claim requires a bit of a historical journey, and this chapter is an important look back into how our children have been propelled into the rabbit hole of living in two worlds, two realities.

Our Amazing Brains and Achievements

Throughout human history our brains have evolved, and each evolutionary change has fostered amazing achievements; human beings have used their brains to make life easier. From Stone Age tools to the wheel, to Gutenberg's printing press and beyond, humanity has excelled at taking nature's raw materials and turning them into whatever made its existence better. For our purposes, let us acknowledge all the advances before the industrial era but focus on the last couple of centuries.

In the 1800s human creativity produced the steam locomotive, photography, the telegraph and telephone and the electric light. The 1900s improved on all those achievements and also saw human beings flying through the air on airplanes, watching television, splitting the atom and making extraordinary advances in medicine such as developing penicillin, eradicating smallpox and mapping the genetic code of human beings, our DNA. However, and despite all of these advances, human existence was still something very much situated in real time with real people.

As the twentieth century progressed, things began to change very quickly. Little things such as vacuum cleaners, cellophane, neon lamps and radio receivers would be overshadowed by Henry Ford's Model T automobile, the first jet engine and the atomic bomb and people walking on the moon. Eventually, our collective ingenuity shifted us from vacuum tubes and transistors into a world of binary code, microchips and digitisation. The World Wide Web arrived along with a growing ability to communicate with people around the world in real time. This, in turn, pried open an expanding virtual universe to adults and children alike. And, eventually, as we entered the twenty-first century, computers became common place in homes and increasingly smaller and transportable.

It is somewhat interesting to note that today's generation of children, adolescents and young adults are often not aware of how markedly different things were for their parents and grandparents, especially in terms of computers and screen devices. The pace at which computers have advanced compared to earlier human endeavours is breathtaking. From the middle of the twentieth century until now, we have made exponential changes to our existence by making computers commonplace. If time travel were possible and you simply went back about 70 years or so you would be able to see that it wasn't until then that computers started to make inroads into modern society. In the early 1950s the first computer language COBOL (Common Business-oriented Language) was developed and was soon followed by FORTRAN (Formula Translation). Try telling today's teenager that there was a time when anyone who wanted to use a computer had to be able to do much more than swipe a finger across a screen and you would likely see eyes rolling in disbelief. Even more alien to them would be the fact that there was a time when a person needed to study and learn to speak the language of the device being used. All that started to change markedly through the intellect and ingenuity of someone by the name of Steve Jobs. Jobs and another computer 'geek' named Steve Wozniak unveiled the first computer with a single circuit board called the Apple I. Computers were still in their infancy and if you are old enough to remember working on a typewriter, then you will likely remember the day word processing became a reality in 1979.

About the time we started processing words instead of type writing them an era of tremendous cultural change began to unfold. The 1980s were huge, or so it seemed. The music industry thrived as did big hair and interesting fashion! Change was everywhere including the tech industry. We were introduced to 'floppy discs', colour computer screen monitors and the first computer to be marketed as a laptop in 1983. And while the global centre for high technology and innovation, Silicon Valley, had been around for some time, this region outside San Francisco grew into social, cultural, technological and financial prominence. Companies began investing heavily in the rapidly growing world of computer technology, while entrepreneurs and research and design departments were working behind the scenes to make computers a household item and ensure the internet was the place to be! By the time the '90s rolled in, much of the Western world was learning to live with, and for, computers. Then in 1993, another technological game changer called the Pentium microprocessor brought graphics and music to another computer level. Things were moving quickly and the dawning of the twenty-first century suggested that things would only accelerate further. However, the world would soon find itself holding its collective breath over an unknown phantom computer menace predicted to spread a swath of destruction and mayhem. Such was the prophecy of something called Y2K.

Looking back, it seems almost comical that with all the advances in technology and the collective brain power of so many intellects and innovators, no one really knew what was going to happen when the binary code of computers would have to shift from years 1999 to 2000. Predictions ranged from planes falling out of the skies to global financial ruin and everything in between due to computers not being able to digitally adapt to a century beginning with the number '2'. As people were preparing to sing Auld Lang Syne and usher in a new century a lingering dread of what was to befall humanity quickly disappeared. Clocks turned over, and January 1, 2000, arrived without incident. The world soon moved on thinking it had dodged a catastrophic digital bullet.

It didn't take long for Y2K to become a distant and farcical memory and fodder for many jokes. The world did not end. Instead, it became ever more available to the masses as Wi-Fi began to take hold of homes and businesses in 2002, making the World Wide Web that much more accessible. Couple this with the emergence of the first widely accessible smartphone in 2007 and much of society would change forever.

A few years after the first smartphones were on the market for consumers, they would become increasingly more affordable and powerful thereby offering children, teens and adults alike access to the world in a handheld device. The technology that once occupied three floors of an IBM building was now available to be held in the palm of our hands. And with this came an ever-expanding universe of websites, 'apps' (applications), blogs and social media. Facebook, Flickr, YouTube, Instagram, Twitter, and later Tik Tok, emerged as part of the cultural zeitgeist and new additions to the English language. Humanity was well and truly into the technological thick of it and the stuff of science fiction for previous generations soon become reality for today's! Perhaps this was when we began to enter the Matrix!

In so far as technological advances, the world has come a long way in a relatively short period of time. Accessing computers with a working knowledge of FORTRAN has given way to swiping access to the world via our fingertips. Moreover, the rather abridged version of events noted above does not even begin to cover the full range of computer and digital ingenuity that has been unleashed. With Artificial Intelligence (AI) also becoming part of our lives in an increasingly rapid way, we can no longer begin to speculate what the future might look like. But we do have some questions!

Of interest to us as researchers, and what should be of interest to parents and educators, is to what extent screen technologies have been superfluous or harmful to each digital generation. The millennials of 2000 have now given way to a more screen-absorbed generation and with each passing day young people are online and on screens more than previous generations. Much of this has happened on our watch and been supported by well-meaning parents and teachers, self-promoting schools, political soundbites and tech companies with a profit margin to consider. Mantras of 'one laptop for every child', or 'iPads for all', have become commonplace for anyone purporting to ensure the best life and scholastic outcomes for today's youth. We think that has come at a cost; such rampant advances have occurred with little scrutiny. Human beings tend to take for granted those things that happen quickly and make life easier. Unfortunately, this has masked some very real issues in terms of the very educational outcomes and wellbeing computers are meant to advance. These are two areas that are worthy of elaboration.

Technology as a Panacea for Learning and 'Schooling'

Schools seem to love computers! By schools we mean the school community at large and in particular, many education bureaucrats, school leaders and teachers. From the time computers started edging their way into people's homes and offices, education systems began to embrace such technologies in schools. Many of you can likely recall the first desktop computers for students in computer labs. For many who were schooled during a time before students had their own devices, computer labs were often a welcome distraction from the everyday realities of classroom endeavour. Now, however, computer labs have passed their use by date and have become a distant memory for most people. Students are often required to bring their own devices and some as young as four are being taught how to 'code'. There seems to be widespread acceptance of computing devices as a must for learners of all ages. What, however, is the current evidence for such claims and what is the current reality in terms of the necessity and utility of computers for learning? We believe these are important considerations, especially given the financial costs of resourcing technology and the dubious claims around the effectiveness and necessity of screen devices.

As noted earlier, and we would agree, computers have revolutionised most aspects of life and work. In educational contexts, computers started making inroads into schools and classrooms from the mid-1970s to their seemingly ubiquitous presence across all school sectors today. Indeed, it would be very difficult not to find some form of information and computer technologies (ICTs) in the hands and/or classrooms of today's students. However, what are the actual costs and benefits of such aspirations and practices? An important consideration given how technology is often presented as a panacea for learning.

First it is our contention that when it comes to computers there is often a taken-for-granted notion that they are necessary and an integral component of learning and academic success. We premise those thoughts given such sentiments are often professed by politicians, ICT specialists, academics and school leaders who more often than not use ICTs as a holy grail for education and often as marketing tools to entice parents into having their children enter "21st century learning". However, our concerns are born out of growing evidence around screens and device use that is worrying and the promotion of such devices as an 'educational must-have' may be complicit in doing more harm than good. We acknowledge that screen devices can be useful tools for some to use but are concerned when the tool appears to be using its owner.

Now you may be thinking the above statements may be alarmist or perhaps the mindful meanderings of a couple of luddites. And before we explore the above ideas further to dispel your critique and further outline any harms associated with screen devices in schools some clarity around our propositions is warranted. Let's start with the reality that we, as researchers and educators acknowledge, admit that identifying screens as the specific 'cause' of any specific adverse event or effect is almost impossible. In research terms this is usually articulated as 'correlation does not equal causation'. For the layperson, this is an important consideration when anyone notes they have various studies or reports that purport to have hard evidence about anything.

If pushed to simplify we would say that correlation basically refers to how some things might be related or show a pattern while causation refers to how something may have directly impacted on something else. For example, there is a positive correlation between height and weight but not height and eye colour. Tall people generally weigh more because they are bigger so a relationship exists but that is not the case for height and eye colour. You can be tall or short and this has no relationship on the colour of your eyes. Causation is less confusing … high temperatures cause people to sweat, exercise causes higher heart rate, lack of oxygen causes death and so on. When it comes to screen devices and any potential harm to young people things get a bit problematic in terms of causation.

If we wanted to substantiate a causal link between time on screens or the consumption of certain screen content we would need to create some kind of experiment to test our hypothesis. And therein lies the problem! Any attempts to conduct an experiment seeking to identify causation whereby a student or group of students might be harmed through such experience is impossible given ethical constraints associated with such research. We can't have an experiment that would result in harm. That is why we believe that whenever anyone speaks of potential risks associated with screens, these are best supported by correlation, not causation; harming students to prove a point is not something any good researcher would attempt, or be allowed to attempt. Relatedly, just because we are unable to randomly assign students to long-term exposure to screens and then measure the degree of harm to various groups does not mean that there are no established negative effects associated with such activities. It is interesting to note, however, that at the time of writing the emergence of studies identifying causal links between the use of, and time on, screens and changes to the developing brain are becoming available.[1] We also hope that the chapters you are now working through will give you further pause to consider that screen devices are likely changing the developing brain in ways we are only beginning to understand but the changes are evident.

As you hold the thought of the potential for screen devices to alter the brains, and by association behaviours, of the young people around us, let us delve into some important contextual considerations around screen use. We will start by exploring those things that are often accepted as a reality, or 'true', when in fact there is little evidence to support them.

[1] See, for example, Hutton et al. (2020); Hutton et al. (2022); Maza et al. (2023).

The Divine Glow of Screens in Schools

The history of all manner of technologies in schools is very diverse and lengthy. Starting from chalk and blackboards to film projectors and overheads, schools have seen their fair share of modern-day advances. In the context of this chapter a prudent exploration of computers in schools originates in the 1980s.

As alluded to earlier, during the '80s, there was a steady increase in personal computer use in homes, businesses and schools. As we like to do, let's begin with some anecdotal history. I (Michael) was a high school student during the '80s and remember the first time I saw a personal computer and heard the hyperbolic concerns around preparing for the future due to advancements in computers and computer technology. As I moved into university, many of my peers were lining up to study the languages of computers. We were told that we had to prepare for a brave new world. The rhetoric around the importance of computers and schooling, not too dissimilar to today's proclamations, was amplified as technology was seen as beneficial for students so that they would be better prepared for the jobs and skills of the future. Equally similar then, were assertions that learning a screen was critical for one's future, a belief that still exists. If we do not provide computers (then) or screen devices (now) and are not engaging children in technology, they will somehow be left behind. After all these years I have never had a cogent description of what being left behind meant but such claims, from the outset seem paradoxical if you think about it. It is likely that most of you have never studied computer programming and yet are quite able to use a computer or smartphone with little difficulty. Even the most senior of our communities are actively doing things on tablets, smartphones and laptops. Two clever social experiments push our scepticism about the utility of screens further.

In 1999, when computers were making inroads into all areas of society, researchers from NIIT (a management training company in India), and under the guidance of Dr Sugata Mitra, carved a 'hole in the wall' that separated the NIIT premises from the adjoining slum in Kalkaji, New

Delhi.[2] Through this hole, the researchers built what looked like a poorly constructed garden shed and made a number of newly modern conveniences available to anyone including a freely accessible computer. This computer proved to be an instant hit among many of the impoverished that lived in the slum, especially the children. While many adults were cautious of, or avoided the computer altogether, the children were far more adventurous. With no prior experience, understanding or instruction, they learnt to use the computer on their own, through trial and error and fuelled by their curiosity. It is important to remember that the computers of the time were far less user friendly than those we use today.

Now let's travel more than a decade forward from the NIIT experiment. In 2012 another social experiment occurred in Ethiopia under the 'One Laptop Per Child' program. This program, founded by Nicholas Negroponte, was being implemented in various countries around the globe. The vision of Negroponte and the program was to enhance global education by putting a cheap laptop in the hands of some of the most poverty-stricken children on earth. One of the most fascinating outcomes of this philanthropic endeavour occurred in 2012 with 20 Ethiopian children aged six and seven.[3] In a similar vein as the NIIT experiment in 1999, representatives from the One Laptop program dropped off closed boxes taped shut and containing small tablets with no instructions to the 20 children noted. Many in the organisation, including Nicholas Negroponte, thought that the children would play with the boxes and ignore the devices inside due to their lack of understanding of the enclosed technology. However, it turned out that within four minutes, one child not only opened the box but also found the on-off switch and powered it up. Within five days, those 20 children were using approximately 47 apps per child, per day. Within two weeks, they were singing ABC songs they had learned on the laptops to their families and friends in the village. Their curiosity unabated, it was also reported that within five months, some children had hacked the android operating framework while switching on the camera systems that had been inadvertently disengaged by members of the One Laptop organisation. Like those children in the

---

[2] Mitra et al. (2005).

[3] Korones (2012).

Indian slums in 1999, and in the absence of any formal instruction, the Ethiopian youngsters demonstrated that their innate curiosity and adventurous spirit were all they needed to get technology working for them.

The two examples offered are not meant to suggest that there isn't a place for ICTs in schools per se, but rather are presented to help contest any notion of a child being left behind if they are not provided with computers in schools. It is important to remember that in both cases, the technology available was not nearly as advanced as it is today. In fact, today's technology is designed to be so user friendly that instruction manuals for phones, tablets and computers are either not provided or offer little more than basic start up and warranty information. Moreover, considering the history of rapid advancement and innovation in all measures of ICT, does anyone seriously believe that teaching coding to four-year-old children, as is the case in many schools today, will be of any use to them in a decade when they turn 14? And let's not forget the seemingly unbridled potential of AI. If Alexis can now turn on our music with a voice command, what might it do as AI expands? These questions may seem a bit flippant but nevertheless important given the financial resourcing of ICTs and growing evidence that technology, and by association computers and the internet, appear to do little in terms of academic outcomes.

Screens, Outcomes and Achievement

Along with claims suggesting the lack of access to ICTs may hinder a student's future and leave them somehow 'behind', there has also been, and continues to be, a sort of unscrutinised zeitgeist purporting ICTs as integral to notions of improving learning, academic skills and outcomes. Since the turn of the century, and increasingly over the past decade, many educational innovators have touted technology as a panacea for learning. Such individuals have been supported by politicians who have placed technology at the forefront of notions of an educational revolution. For example, in 2007, then opposition leader of Australia's federal Labour Party, Kevin Rudd, announced his vision of a digital education revolution (DER) program before the upcoming federal election of the time.

The program would provide every Australian student in Years 9 to 12 with laptops. Moreover, this $1 billion dollar initiative would be further funded to purportedly keep laptop use in schools at the cutting edge of technology. Five years after Rudd's announcement, and after a change in leadership, Prime Minister Julia Gillard maintained that pledge whereby the government spent over $2.1 billion on the laptop program.

That was certainly a financial revolution … and we would like to think that spending more than 3 billion dollars on any education initiative would yield some tangible and measurable benefits, especially in terms of educational outcomes. However, little, if any, data pertaining to such benefits is available. Nor have any successive politicians hailed a further call to educational arms to advance a technological revolution. We do acknowledge that there have been a disparate range of studies across various curriculum and pedagogical areas to find links between monies spent and outcomes achieved with little to show for all the effort. Instead, well-established research findings in the disciplines of cognitive science, human factors and the psychology of learning suggest that ICTs may in fact have a deleterious impact on learning. The following is a bit of a laundry list as to why that might be so.

Let's start with recognising that the sheer volume of information available to students through the use of computers can create cognitive overload. This is likely compounded by deficits in attention with the constant shifting of focus due to how that information is presented; 'pop-ups'; instant messages and alerts from 'apps' make devices inherently distracting. Perhaps one could say computers in school create a Matrix of *inopportunity* for deep and meaningful learning.[4] Such concerns are exacerbated by studies and reports related to the use and potential overuse of technology in terms of the very skills and outcomes many technology enthusiasts suggest are enhanced through ICTs in schools. Considering that almost a decade ago researchers found language and learning deficits in 11 to 18-year-old students who used technology excessively,[5] it should not be surprising that questions related to the efficacy and utility of ICTs in schools have grown. Nowhere is this more apparent than in a special

[4] Wood et al. (2011).

[5] Fried (2008).

report published in 2015 by the Organisation for Economic Co-operation and Development (OECD).[6]

Anecdotally, consider *how* "at your fingertips" technology may have prevented *depth* of learning. Rachael began her original tertiary education in the early 90s—back then as today, one of the more surprising aspects of studying psychology is the relentless training in statistics. Statistics now is taught via a range of software programs (SPSS, Jamovi etc), where the students are instructed on which boxes to tick, and which queries to enter in order to spit out an interpretable figure that appropriately answers a research question. In reality, it's just a matter of telling the software program which parameters to set, and where the goalposts are.

Contrast that to Rachael's original training which (somewhat frustratingly) involved drawing up tables on foolscap paper in an old library, writing down the numbers, using a calculator to apply a range of formulas and then consulting published "cut-off" tables to obtain that same interpretable figure.

Now I'm sure you're all cheering that the former has overtaken the latter (and so is Rachael for that matter!). But herein lies the difference. In "doing" all that mathematical work "by hand", students have a better appreciation of exactly how these numbers are being manipulated, and for what purpose. Ask a stats student today what the sum of squares is for and expect to receive a blank stare. The conceptual understanding behind bashing instructions into a program is largely absent. Sure, it's mildly taught as a theoretical adjunct but at the end of the day most statistics graduates know how to operate the machinery, yet have little idea what's happening behind the scenes. Just like most of us drive a car, but need a mechanic when a strange noise erupts from the engine.

Again, we're not advocating here for a return to an abacus instead of a calculator. The reality is most students/professionals don't *need* a conceptual level of understanding of statistics to engage in their daily activities. They just need to know how to run a sensible analysis from time to time. But it sure does come in handy and is even vital in some circumstances—most especially when understanding published research and being able to truly appreciate what those numbers are actually telling you (or not as the

[6] Organisation for Economic Cooperation and Development (OECD) (2015).

case may be). And this is where Rachael's ancient training comes in handy, when assessing the work of peers as a reviewer, it sure helps to know what those little numbers are truly telling you.

For most who work in education contacts, the OECD is a familiar organisation due to their international assessments of student performance in reading, mathematics and scientific literacy. Conducted every three years, the Programme for International Student Assessment (PISA) tests 15-year-olds across the three domains noted and publishes those findings with the intent to assist governments of participating countries in monitoring educational outcomes against a common framework. In 2015, 72 countries participated in PISA and the findings indicated that *Australia had recorded significant declines* in mathematical literacy since 2003, in scientific literacy since 2006 and in reading literacy since 2009. Overall, Australia has continually dropped in its rankings.[7]

Rankings in Australia are important to many. The ongoing PISA test results fuel political slogans and contentious debates related to those results and what needs to be done. Every time the results are announced the battle call for raising educational standards can be heard in federal and state parliament. We have never come across a good argument for lowering standards so raising them seems self-evident. The questions however, are how do we go about raising standards and what can be contributing to their decline? Afterall, you can't fix something if you don't know where it's broke!

It is important to emphasise that PISA continually receives a great deal of attention and will likely do so after every iteration of tests that take place. When we start to look at how to improve outcomes for Australian students, the silence surrounding the OECD's report on students, computers and learning published in 2015 does not garnish any fraction of attention the test results get. Remember, this report was done by the same organisation whose tests are seen as a gold standard for cross country comparisons and a benchmark for academic achievement.

Students, Computers and Learning: Making the Connection makes for interesting reading, especially when examined in conjunction with PISA findings. The report provides an in-depth analysis of ICT usage in OECD

---

[7] OECD (2023).

countries and the results of this analysis do not present a very positive picture. Consider the following passages from the foreword of the report where Andreas Schleicher, the OECD's Director for Education and Skills notes:

> *... students who use computers very frequently at school do a lot worse in most learning outcomes, even after accounting for social background and student demographics ...*

and that

> *... the results also show no appreciable improvements in student achievement in reading, mathematics and science in the countries that had invested heavily in ICT for education ...*

and finally,

> *... put simply, ensuring that every child attains a baseline proficiency in reading and mathematics seems to do more to create equal opportunities in a digital world than can be achieved by expanding or subsidising access to high-tech devices and services.*[8]

Clearly, the OECD's Director for Education and Skills assertions are worth some consideration given the time and resources spent in ensuring students have access to screens and any claims that screens boost academic outcomes. Some might suggest that the sentiments articulated by Andreas Schleicher can simply be part of an isolated study. To the credit of the OECD, that same report goes on to note that their findings are "remarkably similar to the emerging consensus in the research literature, based on studies that use more rigorously designed evaluations".[9] In other words, the report echoes robust research studies noting that ICTs in school may not be the panacea for learning some would promote as necessary for the future.

---

[8] OECD (2015, pp. 3–4).

[9] Ibid, pp. 162.

The findings of the OECD and related studies as noted above do little to support arguments made by ICT enthusiasts regarding the use of screen devices and academic outcomes. Arguably, those enthusiasts might look at the OECD's findings and drive the 'correlation does not indicate causation' barrow noted earlier as a means of diminishing any negative findings. Interestingly, and perhaps almost prophetically, the OECD's report notes that the most frequent pattern emerging from the data is a weak and sometimes negative association between investment in ICT usage and academic outcomes. Furthermore, that notation also mirrors other empirical studies and evaluations of the efficacy of ICTs in schools. One such evaluation based on 81 meta-analyses of research published over the past 30 years found that, on average, ICT's effect on learning had little, if any impact as compared to other teaching interventions.[10] If all of this information is an accurate representation of the efficacy of ICTs in schools then the ongoing financial costs of promoting and pushing a device for all children or the continued resourcing of the most recent ICT products seems misguided and wasteful. Indeed, the last decade has seen a growing body of research literature concerned with the utility of ICTs in schools. However, any discussion about ICTs in schools needs to go beyond the utility and perceived benefits of devices in classrooms and encompass a broader picture of learning with a particular focus on education's complicity in problems associated with screen devices, mental health and wellbeing.

Screens and Student Wellbeing

Now this book is ostensibly all about the potential adverse effects of screen time on health and wellbeing. So the remainder of this chapter offers a glimpse into that presumption as it pertains to students, wellbeing and using technology in school. However, before looking at some examples of the potential impact of screen devices on student wellbeing, it is important to reiterate the proposition that started this chapter in relation to correlation and causation. It is highly likely that what is

[10] Hattie (2013).

presented below will be critiqued by ICT advocates from all backgrounds as correlational. This is a fair comment but unfounded in its overall veracity and accuracy. Remember, we cannot do experiments that harm students but that does not mean that studies that speak to potential harms can be discounted. Moreover, it is important to consider that educators are bound by the Latin phrase, 'in loco parentis', meaning 'in the place of a parent'. Given the underlying responsibility of that sentiment, teachers, and by association schools, must always bear in mind that they act as parents when at school and as such they must be willing to consider any evidence related to screen usage and student wellbeing. In other words, blindly accepting computers as a necessity for classroom endeavour without looking at bigger picture issues and challenges is arguably not conducive to any notion of acting like a parent and indeed there is a growing list of studies rendering the rampant use of screen devices as problematic.

The range of issues being researched in relation to screen devices and wellbeing is rather expansive as evident in other chapters in this book, all of which get considerable attention. For this chapter, however, we focus on three areas of concern that schools may be contributing to without even realising they are doing so. We then examine some related trends that go beyond the schoolyard. The first of these issues relates to sedentary behaviour.

Sitting is the new smoking! This sentiment has emerged over the last few years to express growing concerns with just how much time people, of all ages, spend sitting at the expense of healthy movement and physical activity. Sedentary behaviour has been linked to a rise of negative health outcomes including obesity and metabolic syndrome. Metabolic syndrome refers to a group of risk factors that increase the likelihood of developing serious health problems, such as heart disease, stroke and diabetes. Therefore we contend that the need for physical activity and exercise is self-evident and does not require a lengthy justification of their merits here. Indeed the benefits of exercise and movement on improving physical health, fighting disease are well documented as is the abundance of research linking regular exercise with reducing the risks of depression, anxiety and the prevention of many other physical and psychological conditions.[11] What is worthy of consideration, however, is the extent to which such activity has diminished over the last couple of decades and one of the contributing factors to that phenomenon—screen time.

As noted above, the links between sedentary behaviour and negative health outcomes are well established. Relatedly, obesity is one of the best-documented outcomes of screen media exposure as a result of sedentary behaviour while screen use appears to be a risk factor for the development of metabolic syndrome in children and adolescents.[12]

Worryingly numerous studies have demonstrated that sedentary behaviour is increasing and highly prevalent in young people. Just prior to the pandemic, global surveillance data showed that half of all children and adolescents spent more than two hours a day in screen-based activities with earlier studies having identified that screen device driven sedentary behaviour accounted for over six hours a day in children and more than seven hours a day in adolescents.[13] It wouldn't be too much of a stretch to assume that the amount of time on screens increased during, and as a result of, the pandemic. As much of the world constrained the movements of people and forced millions into their homes during Covid-19, many of those same people were told to 'pivot' to technology for work and 'schooling'. Children and adults alike were forced to shift from being with others to being alone with others via screens. And while many have returned to their place of work or education, many are still working and/or studying from home.

Life after the pandemic is often described as a 'new' normal and that new normality has witnessed the pre-pandemic trend of children increasing their time on screens and earlier in life as documented throughout this book. For schools we believe that supporting and strengthening the health and wellbeing of children and adolescents alike necessitates replacing screen induced sedentary learning activities with non-screen-based learning activities. A screen device should be a tool to be used from time to time rather than a tool that has students sitting and contributing to a

[11] Hu et al. (2020).

[12] Robinson et al. (2017); Sina et al. (2021).

[13] Konstostoli et al. (2021); see also Thomas et al. (2019).

second concern whereby students are often living a life of distraction as they 'multi-task'.

Multi-tasking in its simplest sense may be defined as doing more than one activity simultaneously. Multi-tasking is not a new phenomenon, but technology has arguably reinvigorated research into this area given its capacity for presenting multiple platforms of information simultaneously. One of the most interesting dilemmas with multi-tasking is that when we try to pay attention to more than one thing at a time, such pursuits increase distractibility and slow performance on tasks due to interference in decision-making or what is known at 'Cognitive Bottleneck'.[14] In simpler terms, having to switch from one task to another is time-consuming, takes effort and often ends in errors. For example, you might respond to emails while listening to a presentation, or finish typing a report or be scrolling through your social media while responding to someone's questions, in the belief that combining two tasks will allow you to complete them sooner than if you did them separately. The problem is that human beings are bad at shifting between different tasks because our thinking is actually limited by our ability to pay attention to our working memory and as such we make mistakes or lose track of what we are actually doing.[15]

Most will understand what it means to pay attention to something. We'd ask that you now pay attention to the following description of working memory. Working memory is the mental space where we do conscious active thinking and that space is very limited in capacity and duration. Everything new that we learn is processed through our working memory before it can be committed to long-term or permanent memory systems. In the end, trying to pay attention to multiple things, which is often the case when using screen devices, and get your working memory to do more than it can negatively impacts learning and decision-making. This is one of the reasons why computers can impair performance, distract learners and lead to frustration. This is especially true when attempts to multi-task become habitual. Moreover, while many students might suggest that they can easily switch back and forth between tasks, the

[14] Borst et al. (2010).

[15] Tombu et al. (2011).

evidence suggests that switching isn't a problem, but refocusing and processing any information is diminished. Only the shallowest of 'learning' is taking place. Coordinating physical activities like playing the piano while singing is one thing but it's another to actually commit any school-related learning activities to long-term memory, especially those that require focused attention and thinking. Many times, less is more.

There is ample evidence to suggest that students who engage in multi-tasking behaviours dramatically increase the time to complete tasks, the number of memory errors committed and the processing time associated with such activities while simultaneously diminishing any learning requiring complex cognitive activity.[16] Finally, while prolonged multi-tasking may interfere with learning in a myriad of ways such activity is only symptomatic of broader challenges associated with screen usage that transcend notions of learning and focus more worryingly on wellbeing.

There are a multitude of studies that have explored a range of problems associated with computer usage, smartphones, video games, social media, the internet and other aspects of technology that we so easily take for granted.[17] Two areas of concern related to wellbeing that schools may be complicit in contributing to are overuse and sleep disturbance. Now you might be thinking that schools do not dictate when a student goes to sleep, but as schools continue to embrace technology it should be self-evident that students will spend more of their waking hours in front of screens in school and elsewhere. Much of this activity is also directly linked to attending to school-related tasks and homework. Concurrently, the overuse of technology can be found across a range of studies and the term addiction has now been linked with various aspects of screen devices.[18]

Screen and internet addiction are a genuine concern for parents, educators and mental health professionals as evident by an increasing number of reports and studies highlighting the potential consequences of overuse. Furthermore, the Diagnostic and Statistical Manual (DSM) of

---

[16] Wood et al. (2011).

[17] See Twenge (2011, 2017) and Haidt (2024) for an expansive and authoritative list of challenges and issues related to screen use, children and adolescents.

[18] Kakabadse et al. (2009).

the American Psychiatric Association, the standard for diagnosing mental health issues, added internet addiction to its most recent edition.[19] Internet addiction is an emergent disorder and while there exists much debate as to the constituent elements and symptoms of this relatively new mental health issue, anecdotal evidence and reports of parents struggling to separate their children from their screens suggests that we should be mindful and watchful of screen time. This is also true of schools that insist on the use of computers during lessons whereby any extra time on screen may be contributing to total daily screen time. As parents and educators we would add that time on screens supposedly devoted to learning is often used for other activities beyond those related to school. It is incredibly easy to shift from 'learning activities' to social media or gaming at the blink of an eye and beyond the gaze of any supervising adult. Finally, and most notably, depending on how much time a student spends on a computer during class time along with the time they spend on personal devices like smartphones during breaks, there is also reason to worry about a lack of social interaction that is vital for wellbeing.

Human beings are social beings! This claim is supported by decades of research telling us that being with other people is a vital component to all measures of development and health. Indeed, if the global pandemic that started in 2019 taught us anything, it is that isolation via lockdowns makes us unwell. Consider that in the early years of life, all aspects of a child's overall development are influenced by social interaction and the intrinsically human need to engage socially permeates adolescent development and most aspects of healthy adult life. Unfortunately, screen devices have had a negative impact on this important component of human endeavour. Face-to-face interaction appears to have begun diminishing due to an increase in computers and electronic media use since 1997 and this gap continues to grow as people engage with screens rather than other people.[20] Worryingly, it appears that heavy ICT use at the intersection of social media may also be contributing to feelings of loneliness and anxiety amongst school-aged children.[21] Equally worrisome is

[19] American Psychiatric Association (2013).
[20] Twenge (2011).
[21] Ibid.; Sigman (2009).

the fact that ICTs may be exacerbating various mental health concerns in young people due to sleep deprivation.

Not unlike the wide swath of research related to the importance of social interaction in terms of human development and human flourishing, there is an equally burgeoning body of research related to social interaction and numerous aspects of physical and mental health and sleep. This is covered in greater detail in the next chapter but is worthy of a bit of foreshadowing here.

It is well-established in the scientific literature that sleep is not only important in terms of all aspects of health and healthy development but also in terms of memory, cognition and learning.[22] As you are working through this chapter and as you go about the business of your day you are storing all kinds of information in your working memory in preparation for long-term storage in regions throughout your brain. What you remember is generally a product of what you actively pay attention to and/or anything that generates a great deal of emotional arousal. However, it is when we are asleep that our brains are busy consolidating our memories.

Sleep is not only an important aspect of memory formation but when we are tired due to lack of sleep our capacity for highly functioning cognitive activity is compromised. Not enough sleep means we may not think as efficiently or clearly as we might like, and this can be further impacted by our emotional state. Not enough sleep often leads to negative emotions and a very unpleasant disposition. This has implications for all levels of child development and schooling. Tired minds do not perform well! This has even greater implications for adolescent students whose sleeping patterns change markedly with the onset of puberty and who appear to be chronically sleep-deprived. For adolescents the onset of sleep happens later than their younger siblings and often later than their parents. Changes to circadian rhythms and the later release of melatonin in the brain to induce sleep as compared to adults, coupled with the need to go to school, extracurricular activities or a part-time job early in the morning means adolescence is the time when the eyes are closed for shorter periods. Paradoxically, adolescence is also the time when the

---

[22] Nagel (2014).

average young person needs at least nine hours of sleep per night. Rhetorically speaking, one might ask how schools play a role in setting sleep times for students and the answer can be found in one word: 'homework'.

Homework, in itself, is a contentious educational phenomenon with much debate around the utility and efficacy of having students do more schoolwork after hours. In terms of screen time, the problem with homework may not necessarily be homework per se, but more specifically the guidelines for submitting homework. It is now common practice for schools to provide online submission of assignments coupled with dubious timelines for such submissions; midnight is not an uncommon deadline for handing in assignments! Placing these types of parameters around the submission of homework sets students up for even greater sleep disturbances. Most people are aware that the blue light emitted from computers and handheld devices has been shown to suppress the production of melatonin, elevate states of arousal and, by association, negatively impact on sleep patterns and behaviour. Again, as parents and educators we feel fairly confident in also noting that many adolescents leave things to the last minute to complete. Couple this with issues around potentially being less efficient in completing a task due to notions of multi-tasking discussed earlier and homework is often submitted later rather than sooner. If this is indeed midnight, then the total time for restful sleep is greatly diminished.

Finally, given that adolescents, tend to be chronically sleep deprived, it is noteworthy that a recent study of school-aged children in Canada found that losing just one hour of sleep negatively impacted on short-term memory, emotional functioning, attention, working-memory and academic performance.[23] As noted earlier, there is plenty of evidence telling us that sleep is essential for children to function productively and get the most out of each day.

We hope that by now you can see that the glowing light of technology in the lives of children may not be very divine! Screens have made inroads in schools and indeed contributed much to the collective lives of children and adults alike. However we are only beginning to see that

[23] Hayes and Bainton (2020); see also Newbury et al. (2021); Yang et al. (2022a, 2022b).

what screens provide may not be entirely positive. Could it be that screens are metaphorically creating a generation of Neos longing to find their way around their own Matrix? And for those who have not seen the film or have forgotten its antagonists, sentient machines known as 'Agents' are set out to destroy Neo and his comrades in an effort to stop humans from escaping the Matrix. Let us hope that we are not too late. Moreover, if this chapter wasn't enough to convince you, but perhaps the next chapter will give you further pause for thought and a growing determination for helping students thrive in a real world rather than getting lost in a virtual one. Being alone together, or forever elsewhere in a virtual matrix is not conducive to human flourishing!

Summary

The chapter above investigated how screen technology has fundamentally altered human reality, drawing parallels to the film "The Matrix" where humans navigate dual realities. It critically assessed many educational system's embrace of digital technologies, challenging the assumption that computers inherently improve learning outcomes. Evidence from OECD reports and research studies suggests minimal or negative correlations between heavy ICT investment and academic achievement. The chapter also explored three key concerns related to screen usage: increased sedentary behaviour among children, diminished cognitive performance from multi-tasking, and disruptions to sleep patterns and social development. Despite significant financial investment in classroom technology, research indicates these devices may contribute to poorer academic outcomes and compromised wellbeing. Questions around whether educational technology initiatives represent worthwhile investments or whether they inadvertently contribute to developmental issues in young people are also interrogated. In the end the research provided advocates for a more balanced approach that views screen devices as occasional tools rather than educational necessities, enabling students to thrive in genuine human interaction rather than becoming immersed in a digital matrix.

Bibliography and Further Reading

American Psychiatric Association (2013). *Diagnostic and Statistical Manual of Mental Disorders (DSM-5) – 5th Edition.* American Psychiatric Association Publishing.

Borst J.P., Taatgen, N. A. & van Rijn, H. (2010). The problem state: a cognitive bottleneck in multitasking. *Journal of Experimental Psychology, Learning, Memory and Cognition*, 36(2), 363–82. https://doi.org/10.1037/a0018106. PMID: 20192536.

Fried, C. B. (2008). In-class laptop use and its effects on student learning. *Computers & Education*, 50(3), 906–914.

Haidt, J. (2024). *The Anxious Generation: How the Great Rewiring of Childhood is Causing an Epidemic of Mental Illness.* Allen Lane.

Hattie, J. (2013). *Visible Learning and the Science of How We Learn.* Routledge, London.

Hayes, B. &Bainton, J. (2020) The impact of reduced sleep on school related outcomes for typically developing children aged 11–19: A systematic review. *School Psychology International*, 41(6), 569–594. https://doi.org/10.1177/0143034320961130

Hu, S., Tucker, L., Wu, C. & Yang, L. (2020). Beneficial effects of exercise on depression and anxiety during the Covid-19 pandemic: A narrative review. *Frontiers in Psychiatry*, 11:587557. https://doi.org/10.3389/fpsyt.2020.587557

Hutton, J.S., Dudley, J., Horowitz-Kraus, T., DeWitt, T. & Holland, S.K. (2020). Associations between screen-based media use and brain white matter integrity in preschool-aged children. *JAMA Pediatrics*, 174(1), e193869. https://doi.org/10.1001/jamapediatrics.2019.3869.

Hutton, J.S., Dudley, J., DeWitt, T. & Horowitz-Kraus, T. (2022). Associations between digital media use and brain surface structural measures in preschool-aged children. *Scientific Reports*, 12, 19095. https://doi.org/10.1038/s41598-022-20922-0

Kakabadse, A.P., Kakabadse, N.K., Bailey, S. & Myers, A. (2009). *Techno Addicts: Young Person Addiction to Technology,* Sigel Press.

Kontostoli, E., Jones, A.P., Pearson, N., Foley, L., Biddle, S.J.H. & Atkin, A.J. (2021). Age-related change in sedentary behavior during childhood and adolescence: A systematic review and meta-analysis.

Korones, S. (2012). Ethiopian kids teach themselves using only tablet computers. www.zdnet.com/article/ethiopian-kids-teach-themselves-using-only-tablet-computers.

Maza, M.T., Fox, K.A. & Kwon, S. (2023). Association of habitual checking behaviours on social media with longitudinal functional brain development. *JAMA Pediatrics*, 177(2), 160167. https://doi.org/10.1001/jamapediatrics.2022.4924.

Mitra, S., Dangwal, R., Chatterjee, S., Jha, S., Bisht, R.S. & Kapur, P. (2005). Acquisition of computer literacy on shared public computers: Children and the 'hole in the wall'. Australasian Journal of Educational Technology, 21(3), 407–426. https://doi.org/10.14742/ajet.1328

Nagel, M.C. (2014). *In the Middle: The Adolescent Brain, Behaviour and Learning.* Australian Council for Educational Research (ACER).

Newbury, C.R., Crowley, R., Rastle, K. & Tamminen, J. (2021). Sleep deprivation and memory: Meta-analytic reviews of studies on sleep deprivation before and after learning. *Psychological Bulletin*, 147(11), 1215–1240. https://doi.org/10.1037/bul0000348.

Organisation For Economic Cooperation and Development (OECD) (2015). *Students, Computers and Learning: Making the Connection*. OECD Publishing, Paris, France. https://doi.org/10.1787/9789264239555-en

OECD (2023). *PISA 2022 Results (Volume I): The State of Learning and Equity in Education*, PISA, OECD Publishing. https://doi.org/10.1787/53f23881-en.

Robinson, T.N., Banda, J.A., Hale, L., Lu, A.S., Fleming-Milici, F., Calvert, S.L. & Wartella, E. (2017). Screen media exposure and obesity in children and adolescence. *Pediatrics*, 140 (Suppl2), S97–S101. https://doi.org/10.1542/peds.2016-1758K

Sigman, A. (2009). Well connected?: The biological implications of 'social networking'. *The Biologist*, 56(1), 14–20.

Sina, E., Buck, C., Veidebaum, T. et al (2021). Media use trajectories and risk of metabolic syndrome in European children and adolescents: The IDEFICS/I. Family cohort. *International Journal of Behavioral Nutrition and Physical Activity*, 18(134). https://doi.org/10.1186/s12966-021-01186-9

Thomas, G., Bennie, J.A., DeCocker, K., Castro, O. & Biddle, S.J.H. (2019). A descriptive epidemiology of screen-based devices by children and adolescents: A scoping review of 130 surveillance studies since 2000. *Child Indicators Research*, 13(3), 935–950. https://doi.org/10.1007/s12187-019-09663-1

Tombu, M.N., Asplund, C.L., Dux, P.E., Godwin, D., Martin, J.W. & Marois, R. (2011). A Unified attentional bottleneck in the human brain. *Proceedings of the National Academy of Sciences*, 108(33), 13426–13431. https://doi.org/10.1073/pnas.1103583108

Twenge, J.M. (2011). Generational differences in mental health: Are children and adolescents suffering more or less? *American Journal of Orthopsychiatry*, 81(4), 469–472. https://doi.org/10.1111/j.1939-0025.2011.01115.x

Twenge, J.M. (2017). *iGen: Why Today's Super-Connected Kids Are Growing Up Less Rebellious, More Tolerant, Less Happy – and Completely Unprepared for Adulthood.* Atria Books.

Wood, E., Zivcakova, L., Gentile, P., Archer, K., De Pasquale, D. & Nosk, A. (2011). Examining the impact of off-task multi-tasking with technology on real-time classroom learning. *Computers & Education*, 58(1), 365–374.

Yang, N., Weizhen, X. & Wang, Z. (2022a). Effects of sleep duration on neurocognitive development in early adolescents in the USA: A propensity score matched, longitudinal, observational study. *The Lancet Child & Adolescent Health*, 6(10), 705–712. https://doi.org/10.1016/S2352-4642(22)00188-2.

Yang, N., Liu, T.T. & Wang, Z. (2022b). Functional connectome mediates the association between sleep disturbance and mental health in preadolescence: A longitudinal mediation study, *Human Brain Mapping*, 43, 2041–2050. https://doi.org/10.1002/hbm.25772

4

Screens Are Changing the Brains of Children and Teens: And Not in a Good Way

…all of us at various times in our lives believe true things for poor reasons, and false things for good reasons, and that whatever we think we know, whether we're right or wrong, arises from our interactions with other human beings. There is no truth, only perception.
—Professor Alan Jacobs (2017, p. 39)

Abstract This chapter explores the concerning relationship between excessive screen time and neurodevelopmental outcomes in children and adolescents. Emerging research suggests that "Intensive Early Screen Exposure" correlates with autism-like behaviours, with studies showing that 1–2 hours of screen time at age one doubles the risk of ASD diagnosis by age three. The neurological mechanism for this appears linked to disrupted development of critical social skills, particularly Theory of Mind—the ability to understand others' perspectives. When screens displace real-world social interactions during sensitive developmental periods, children fail to build essential neural pathways for emotional recognition and social reciprocity. This parallels historical cases of severe social deprivation, like Genie Wiley, who demonstrated irreversible developmental deficits. The documented 17-fold increase in ASD diagnoses over 50 years, doubling in the last 20,

M. C. Nagel, R. Sharman, *Virtual Autism and Other Screen Disorders*, Palgrave Studies in Cyberpsychology, https://doi.org/10.1007/978-3-032-00803-9_4

coincides with widespread screen technology adoption. The research noted in the chapter suggests that these trends may also contribute to increasing narcissism, declining empathy, and rising social polarisation observed in younger generations.

Keywords Deprivation of stimulation • Autism Spectrum Disorder (ASD) • Socio-emotional development • Theory of mind • Sensitive periods • Narcissism

Anyone who can remember a world without Facebook and other social media environments would be correct in thinking that there is something strange going on with "young people these days". It is important, however, that must remind ourselves that older generations historically despair at what they see as faults in the younger. However, the generation of Millennials and younger are participating in an interesting experiment, in that they are the first to have developed their growing brains in an increasingly hybrid world of reality and online environments. Remember too, from earlier chapters, that a maturing brain wires itself via stimulation from the environment across many years and reconstructs itself to become more efficient.

To emphasise these important points it is critical to keep this in the back of your mind. The brain isn't fully developed for almost three decades and along with a lengthy period of building its neural superhighway, the brain also refines itself and "prunes" away unnecessary connections. This pruning process coincides with the onset of puberty and continues into our mid-twenties. Most of the action, however, happens in the teenage years as the brain works hard to create a more refined and efficient neural network. The result is that the brain leaves only those connections useful for survival and functioning within its particular social and cultural milieu.

The capacity for the brain to do this sculpting has allowed human beings to adapt and thrive in very different environments and populate regions where other creatures cannot survive. You won't find any polar bears in any desert, but you will find humans living in the Arctic and the Sahara. No other species can do this!

The amazing plasticity of the human brain to develop and adapt to the conditions around it can also be applied to our social skills. As infants we learn very quickly how to get a reaction from our parents (crying, smiling) and as we grow our social skills are formed through reciprocal relationships with others. Just to be clear, there is no disputing that we develop our social skills via interactions with others and there are decades of research to support this. Deprive a child of this stimulation and the end results are not good. The tragic story of Genie Wiley offers a good example.

On November 4, 1970, and purely by chance, a social worker discovered a 13-year-old girl who, by all accounts, had been forcefully deprived of much of the stimulation we have spoken about and that most children and adults take for granted. You see, sometime around 18 months of age this young girl was confined to a small room, not much larger than a closet and often tied to a 'potty' chair. Genie, as she was to be called by social workers to help protect her identity, lived most of her life in extreme deprivation. She was not allowed to speak to anyone including her mother and brother who rarely left the family home and were also forbidden to speak to Genie. Authorities also discovered that on some nights Genie was bound in a sleeping bag and forced to sleep in an enclosed crib with metal screening all around it; in essence a 'chicken wire' jail. Genie grew up isolated from others and with no regular verbal, social or emotional stimulation.

By the age of 13, when she was discovered, Genie was almost entirely mute. In reading this you, like those who discovered her, would probably not be surprised in knowing that she had severe emotional difficulties and limited capacity to communicate with oral language. What did surprise researchers was her physical stature which for all intents and purposes was stunted; she looked more like an eight-year-old than a teenager. Genie was promptly removed from her home and her parents charged with child abuse.

Why her father did this will always remain a mystery as he took his own life before the trial and never explained his actions to anyone including his wife. Genie's mum Irene would later have her charges of abuse dropped. She was deemed a recipient of abuse as well and not complicit in what happened to Genie. What is not a mystery is the profound impact

Genie's environment had on her. She received extensive treatments and therapeutic interventions, but the damage was mostly irreversible. She did progress with basic skills and learned to dress herself and use a toilet but here communication skills never went much further than learning a few new words and speaking in two-word phrases. She was never able to grasp any measure of functional grammar. Genie was returned to her mother in 1975 and eventually ended up in several foster homes due to her mother's incapacity for providing adequate care.

The discovery of Genie presented a unique opportunity for researchers. The opportunity was unique because there was, and is, no way that any experiment could be designed, and gain ethical clearance, in which a child is deliberately deprived of the basic necessities of life in the interests of science. Her discovery provided an opportunity to see the impact of the deprivation of stimulation and whether anything negative could be healed or reversed. Her discovery also supports much of our discussion on how the brain is shaped and adapts to the environment around it during childhood.

The same notions of adaptability can be applied to the social skills well into adolescence. Adolescence is the time where the over-emotional and somewhat reckless brain kicks into full gear to develop peer relationships that will drive future romantic pairings, and hopefully form the basis of a new generation of thinkers and leaders. A key question, then, is what happens in the developing brains of children and young people when those social skills are forming online and/or deprived of real 'in time' face-to-face interactions? The true answer is, we don't yet know. But we have some recent research that gives us cause for concern.

Before we unpack some recent findings, we'd like you to consider the work of Dr Edward Tronick. Dr Tronick is one of the world's leading authorities on child development and the brilliant mind behind what has become known as the "Still Face Experiment". In his work, he and his colleagues created a scenario where a mother and infant are engaging in normal reciprocal interactions; making faces, smiling, playing peek-a-boo and so on. At a point in time the mother turns her head away from the child and then returns her gaze back to the infant, but with a significant change; she keeps her face still with no facial gestures and no interactions with the infant. What happens next is the infant invariably becomes increasingly anxious and stressed by a non-responsive and expressionless mother. They work harder to get mum to engage and make repeated attempts to get the interaction into the usual reciprocal pattern they are used to. When the attempts fail, the infant grows wary, distressed and withdraws with a hopeless facial expression often resulting in tears. Tronick's work remains one of the most replicated findings in developmental psychology. It has been used to demonstrate the importance of attachment and pair-bonding between infants and mothers across cultures. For us, Tronick's work offers yet another example of what can happen when 'normal' reciprocal interactions are interrupted if only for a couple of minutes. Couple this with the tragic story of Genie noted above and we hope you get the picture; depriving children of normal healthy interactions robs them of opportunities to build important social and emotional neural pathways.

Screens and 'Autistic-Like Behaviours'

It should be clear from the points above that 'being' with others is an important component of healthy development. Worryingly, recent times studies are providing troubling concerns related to screens displacing normal interactions and thereby depriving children of the necessary stimulation being discussed here. For example, recently published research in Pediatrics demonstrated higher television/video exposure and less in-real-life play placed one-year-olds (that's right—we're talking about babies here) at greater risk of displaying "ASD-like symptoms".[1] They asked parents fairly basic questions about their infants abilities such as "Does your child look you in the eye", "Does your child ever pretend", " Does your child imitate you", "Does your child sometimes stare at nothing and wander with no purpose", " Does your child seem oversensitive to noise" and so on and so forth. Even in the first year of life, over-exposure to screens and under-exposure to in-real-life interactions made these little one-year-olds "resemble" toddlers with autism.

[1] Kushima et al. (2022).

Not to be outdone by the researchers above, Yalda Uhls had earlier sounded the warning on this possible developmental trajectory where 'normal'.[2] Pre-teens had screens removed for five days while at nature camp. Compared to controls, removing screen time from pre-teens for barely a week, markedly increased their social interaction skills and improved their non-verbal recognition skills—something that cannot occur in those with genuine ASD. So what then is 'ASD'?

Autism Spectrum Disorder is a neurodevelopmental disorder that is often characterised as being on a continuum. Across this continuum we see a range of behaviours from deficits in social communication, restricted interests and fixations on certain activities along with repetitive behaviours. Quite often there is a component of intellectual impairment as well, but that is not always the case. For example, on one end of the continuum, those with profound autism may not speak or be minimally verbal with a low IQ and present many challenges requiring help with the daily tasks of life. On the other end of that same continuum may be some of your colleagues or university-bound students who have unusual talents or abilities but struggle with social and cultural mannerisms. Such a person was depicted masterfully by the actor Jim Parsons in his portrayal of the annoying yet much adored Sheldon Cooper on the TV sitcom, The Big Bang Theory.

There is a great deal of technical aspects around ASD that are worth noting. First, and contrary to popular belief, ASD, is at best, moderately heritable. Most causal hypotheses favour gene by environment interactions, which is a fancy way of saying both nature and nurture interact in equal measure to produce this outcome. Precisely what part of nurture or environment influences the development of ASD remains largely unknown.

Second, While ASD has no doubt been part of the human condition since day dot, diagnosis of ASD has risen from less than 1 per 1000 in the 1960s to 16.8 per 1000 today. Prevalence doubled between 2000 and 2018, although the ratio of males to females remains stable across time at approximately 4:1.[3]

---

[2] Uhls et al. (2014).

[3] Heffler et al. (2020).

Now we'd like you to pause here and just consider the implication of the previous paragraph. ASD diagnoses have exploded 17-fold in the last 50 years doubling in the last 20 years alone. This is a very interesting consideration given something else that has exploded in prevalence; since 2007 the use of smartphones and other screen devices has grown exponentially. We think this important given that it is highly unlikely that DNA or any other predisposing biological influences have shifted that suddenly for nature to play a role in the increasing numbers of individuals on the continuum; as simply put, evolution doesn't work that quickly. The rise of ASD is an avalanche occurring at what should normally be glacial pace. So, neuropsychologists and scientists have been pondering what, in our day-to-day environment, could have shifted so suddenly to cause such an upswing in diagnosis. A common denominator is the omnipotence of screen devices in the hands of young and old alike. And whilst it is fair that awareness and more sensitive detection tools may be responsible for detecting some level of increase, 17-fold in the last 50 years with a doubling in the last 20 cannot be accounted for by a mere moving of diagnostic goal posts.

Another interesting and curious observation related to ASD over the last ten years is the emergence of increasing case reports involving children exposed to what has now been labelled as "Intensive Early Screen Exposure" (over 4 hours per day) that seems to result in "autism-like symptoms" or indeed diagnosis of ASD itself.

Romanian psychologist Marius Zamfir was one of the first to document the increase of autistic-like behaviours in children in relation to intensive early screen exposure (IESE). In 2018 he coined the term "Virtual Autism" after tracking his child patients over a five-year period. To summarise his approach, Zamfir took children referred to him for treatment for autism, kicked them off screens for a minimum of three months, and trained their parents in reciprocal, interactive play (recall the still face experiment and what happens when you deprive a child of reciprocal interactions). After this seemingly simple intervention, a proportion of those children showed such a remediation of autism symptoms, they no longer qualified for the diagnosis at all.

Specifically, improvements were seen in social facial expression, attention/interest towards people, improved language and reduced hyperactivity. Zamfir's work has since been replicated by other researchers around the world.

By 2019, enough high-quality studies had been conducted to allow for a scientific review of the current research by that date, which identified a clear link between screen time and ASD, with authors concluding more research was needed to understand the causal mechanisms.[4] That didn't stop a child psychiatrist writing for Trends in Neuroscience to call for the recognition of a causal link between IESE and ASD, citing challenge-dechallenge-rechallenge research. What this means is when screens were removed from children demonstrating autistic behaviours those behaviours desisted. However, when screens were introduced, the autistic behaviours returned.[5] It is also noteworthy that symptoms of ASD behaviours worsened in children who did have a genuine clinical diagnosis of ASD in response to extended screen time; in other words, their autism got worse![6]

By 2020 research was building citing relationships between screen time and "autism-like behaviours" in babies as young as 12 months of age. In 2022 a particularly strong longitudinal study from Japan, tracking over 80,000 mother-baby dyads demonstrated that 1–2 hours of screen time at age one doubled risk of diagnoses of ASD by age three; 3–4 hours at age one trebled that risk by age three in males.[7]

It doesn't take a PhD level scientist to see what is going on here. And the research just keeps coming—the link between screen time and autism symptoms/diagnostic risk is now clear, and with further longitudinal research will soon be irrefutable. The question this raises for those of us with a scientific bent is: How? It's one thing to describe associations, quite another to deduce what might be happening to cause them.

---

[4] Baio et al. (2018).

[5] Slobodin et al. (2019).

[6] Harle (2019).

[7] Dong et al. (2021).

One way of thinking about this is by casting your mind back to the first two chapters of this book—this is where all that knowledge becomes important. You may remember that the human brain essentially wires itself to the environment in which it finds itself. It is a changing organ, responsive to what it assumes is important for survival. Practically speaking, and according to one of the world's leading researchers on the developing brain, Professor Jay Giedd, this means:

> *If an adolescent is doing music, sports or academics, those are the connections that will be hard wired. If they're lying on the couch or playing video games or watching MTV, those are the cells and connections that are going to survive.*[8]

In terms of what screens could be doing to the developing brain to produce symptoms or a diagnosis of ASD, we already have some candidate brain regions cropping up in the research. Higher screen use has been found to result in lower myelination and organisation of brain white matter tracts that underpin language and cognitive skills. Think of myelin as the plastic coating around electrical wiring. It acts as an insulator and conductor, helps signals transmit quickly to their desired location, and prevents wires from getting crossed. Essentially those regions important for language and cognitive skills if not properly myelinated, will be slow and risk malfunctioning and as such may present as characteristics of ASD.[9] Our sense of the emerging research at the intersection of children and teens spending increasingly high numbers of hours on screens is that we will see even greater evidence of structural, and by association functional, changes to the developing brain.

All of this should raise alarm bells, however, we also know that there are interventions that might counteract the impact of screens. For example, lifelong exposure to green spaces has demonstrated associations with increased grey matter in regions associated with better working memory and attention.[10] From a clinical standpoint this is probably more important in the ADHD context rather than ASD, but you get the picture.

[8] Giedd (2001).

[9] Hutton et al. (2020).

[10] Dadvand et al. (2018).

Relatedly, when we dissect the interventions proposed by Zamfir, digital detox and parental training for two months altered EEG patterns in the brain.[11]

The important take-home message from these brain-based studies is that the brain changes itself in response to environmental stimuli—*experiences matter!* This has been well known for decades, but perhaps neuroscientists were unprepared for just how much nurture could alter the developmental trajectory of the brain. Green spaces, time off screens and positive interactions with parents and peers promote healthy development. Screen time, however, may be poisoning the potential of a developing human being.

There are now a smorgasbord of individual research studies demonstrating a link between screen usage and 'autistic-like behaviours'. And the results should come as no surprise. If you displace real-life activities that build social learning and interpersonal skills with shallow yet entertaining screen-based dopamine hits, you are unlikely to develop the social sophistication required to navigate real-life interactions. Simply stated, screen time is heroin for the mind, and in particular those challenging emotion recognition skills that form the basis of non-verbal communication, are failing to develop.

Screens, Emotions and Navigating Life

The knock-on effects of stunted emotion recognition ability are yet to be fully realised. However, it seems reasonable to speculate that friendship-formation, building strong social bonds and essentially playing well with others would be negatively affected. In the end many aspects of wellbeing are likely to be diminished as children struggle to form and maintain the types of social connections necessary to act as a buffer to mental ill-health. *The Lancet*, a prestigious medical journal confirmed what we've all seen anecdotally, that mental wellbeing in adolescents has "declined

[11] Sadeghi et al. (2021).

considerably during past decades" and noted evidence of detrimental impacts of screen time on mental wellbeing that started at just 1 hour per day.[12]

Mental health is one thing, but we'd also like you to just pause and consider non-verbal recognition skills, because we will be coming back to this point later. Verbal dialogue makes up a maximum of 10% of what we express in any one interaction while body language, facial expressions, posture, possibly even pheromones give away far more. It's no wonder secret agents are specifically trained to recognise "microexpressions". So just think about that for a minute—what happens when you are missing 90% of what's being said? You've just put yourselves in the shoes of a person with autism. People with ASD have enormous trouble discerning anything other than direct verbal or written statements (and often even those as well). Hence their tendency to take everything literally. They can miss sarcasm, jokes, and especially misconstrue a situation where what is said doesn't match the actual feeling behind it (e.g., she smiled with gritted teeth). As one of our mature age students with ASD commented—"imagine walking into a room and everyone is wearing the same face mask. That's all I see, I don't know what they're thinking until they start speaking. And even then, I get into trouble because I think I'm going along with a joke … and then I get the punch to the head".

Aside from intentional punches to the head, so many of our daily interactions are largely intuitive, and those of us raised in-real-life now take for granted our second-nature emotion recognition skills. But these were not with us a birth, they were shaped and honed, as our neurons were pruned and tuned to better discern what was really going on with other people around us. This taken-for-granted process of emotional development is necessary for us to become mentally healthy and socially functioning human beings and plays a role in so much of what we do, especially in terms of relationships. Friendship formation, for example, relies on intimacy-building; the capacity to understand and honestly reciprocate another's interest in you. This is what relationship researchers sometimes call "connection" or "chemistry". Imagine the fall-out if you

[12] Khan et al. (2021).

keep getting this wrong, sometimes even causing inadvertent offence. Far fewer friends for a start.

The outcomes presented in relation to the research linking screen time and deficits in socio/emotional development and process also has links to what is referred to as the Displacement hypothesis—quite simply, while someone is attached to their phone—what ***aren't*** they doing? If we were to use a physical analogy, if you engaged in sedentary behaviour for long periods of time, day after day, we would expect your muscles to weaken, slacken and in extreme cases wither away (office workers, gamers), compared to a person who lives and works using large muscle groups daily (concreter, gym trainer etc.). Similar processes apply to the brain, those connections that are not used or "exercised" weaken and wither away. Again, Genie and the 'Still Face Experiment' provide food for thought.

All of these are especially important considerations during neurodevelopmentally critical or sensitive periods. Consider the baby in the pram on the smartphone. What they aren't doing is looking at the people around them, smiling and trying to get attention, observing the faces and behaviours of the humans in their immediate vicinity. Yet all of these simple interactions are vital for learning. And this is only the beginning. The children at home on devices rather than outside in groups playing with their peers. Adolescents gaming instead of "hanging out" with friends and developing ever increasingly sophisticated social skills.

Let us now move to the crux of the issue—while children are on smartphones or being babysat by screens, what aren't they developing from a cognitive point of view? Here we'd like to take you back to Theory of Mind discussed in earlier chapters. Here's a test we give our students every year—we ask our students, "Does my bum look big in this?"

Now before you leap on the phone to report us to the Dean, the point of this question is to get students thinking—what are we *REALLY* asking? Here are some of the answers we get most years:

- We're asking for reassurance and/or validation,
- We want to know that we are appreciated or liked,
- We're doing some measure of checking perceptions of ourselves to see if they are consistent with other's points of view,

- We're trying to ascertain if we're still seen as attractive or handsome or whether we are appropriately dressed for the occasion,
- We might also be looking for some affirmation related to our overall level of attractiveness, our age or whether our style of clothing suits us or is 'on trend'.

Hilariously, only at the end of a robust discussion do students come to the conclusion that we might, in fact, want an honest opinion! This is the power of ToM—in every human interaction, we are working to figure out what the other person is REALLY trying to communicate, and how to best respond. At its simplest, ToM is the understanding that people have different mental representations, thoughts and feelings. So just because I prefer coffee to tea, I don't assume that everyone else does. So, I would ask people visiting me what refreshment they would prefer.

Up until about the age of three or four years, most children haven't developed a terribly sophisticated ToM. They honestly believe that whatever they think, feel or see, is what everyone else thinks, feels or sees. Have you ever had that funny moment when your young child plays hide and seek for the first time—and instead of concealing themselves, they cover their eyes? Hence "hiding" means covering their own eyes, because surely if they can't see, neither can you!

Poorly developed ToM also explains a lot about the terrible two tantrums. Imagine a two-year-old is thirsty, but for some unknown reason you aren't offering them a drink! Why not? You should know they're thirsty because at this age they earnestly believe they belong to a hive mind. So, they whinge, cry and maybe even throw a tantrum, because they are not happy with the fact that you aren't giving them what they want! Eventually this frustration gives way to understanding that they actually need to communicate their needs to you, via gesture or speech. As they experiment with this amazing revelation, the explosion in language and communication at this age begins.

As we move through the terrible twos and well into adulthood, our ToM is one of the rare functions that continues to improve with age. It becomes increasingly sophisticated as we encounter more and more social situations (including complex and awkward ones such as flirting, lying or cheating) and we learn about our societal expectations of our response.

ToM also underpins imagination (putting yourself in another's shoes, or a hypothetical scenario), perspective-taking, friendship formation and even age-old wisdom. It should come as no revelation to know that ToM is of course, the function most impaired in autism.

Although ASD lists symptoms (poor socio-emotional communication; repetitive and restricted interests), it is impairment in the underlying ToM that gives rise to these behaviours. Lack of ToM is catastrophic for perspective-taking ability; which brings with it disinterest or poor development in language development, emotion recognition and reciprocity in interactions. This is why some people with ASD can become socially tedious as they talk on and on about their own interests (repetitive and restricted interests) with little interest in anything anyone else has to say. And to be fair, they're not trying to be rude, they probably just aren't picking up your social/emotional signals that you are bored or frustrated with the conversation. And if they have little intrinsic interest in you or your hobbies—why go through the effort of starting a conversation about it?

At the more serious end of the spectrum, some readers may be musing that ASD "meltdowns" share some similarities with two-year-old tantrums (except in a post-pubescent large body this can be downright dangerous). To be fair toddler tantrums and meltdowns are a simplistic comparison, but there is something to consider that if your needs weren't being met, coupled with you having no way of communicating them, and then attributing that to malice on those around you failing to respond the way you want, dear reader you may well engage in an adult tantrum in that circumstance as well.

Poorly developed ToM (whether you are autistic or not) will have significant implications for your ability to navigate a range of social situations, develop empathy for those you disagree with, understand the motives and perspectives of others, and ultimately build positive and long-lasting bonds with other people.

As we noted earlier, whilst ToM will erupt seemingly quite suddenly around the age of three–four, it continues to improve with age due to experience. Experience, practice, making mistakes and learning from trickier and trickier social situations. So, we ask you to reflect on our earlier question: whilst children are glued to their phones, what social activities are they not undertaking that are important for this vital brain function? Relatedly, an inability to understand another's perspective, which has become another defining feature of younger generations, can create numerous problems, especially when it comes to relationships. And we do know that rates of ASD are rising along with the behaviours and challenges associated with this phenomenon. Could this be one of the reasons why the United Kingdom now has a Minister for "Loneliness"? Hardly surprising in a world where people are becoming less equipped to build and maintain friendships, because they simply lack the learned ability to do so.

Notwithstanding the challenges associated with evidence noting a decline in abilities in perspective-taking, researchers who have been studying generational changes are also noting some consistent patterns. The generational decline in perspective-taking ability parallels a generational increase in narcissism. This is thought to be due, in some part at least, to a shift of values away from community and social affiliations to money, fame and image; think 'likes', being 'followed' or 'trending' and being an 'influencer'. Narcissism is, arguably, not a positive attribute and declines in prosocial behaviour and less civic engagement (interest in social issues, government, and politics) further reduces the opportunity for social connections that build perspective-taking.

An inability to make social connections and friends along with increases in narcissism requires us to consider what might be contributing to such worrying phenomenon. Research has found some support that social media has impacted perspective-taking due to the digital algorithms that foster confirmation and form online siloes where we only see and hear from people who think the same as we do. Whistleblower Frances Haugen confirmed that Facebook was little more than an echo chamber that deliberately sent polarising information to solidify already-held views and promote in-group/out-group thinking.[13] So imagine a teen sitting at their computer, whipping themselves into a frenzy about the latest social issue—fed by the algorithms of Facebook to dumb down any alternative perspective lest it lead to some critical thinking, or heaven forbid,

[13] Fitzsimmons (2023).

empathy for another's position. One could even suggest that this is a form of 'personal fake news'!

This inability to "tolerate" another's point of view, ironically in a generation that likes to trot out "inclusivity" and "diversity" at every virtue signalling opportunity, has led to some spectacular fallouts. Being the old fogeys we are, we remember with a sense of bewildered bemusement the fracture caused in the UK during the "Brexit" vote. Now neither of us have any expert understanding of the issues between the EU and UK, but what was of interest to us was the impact at ground level of this debate on everyday families. Young people started to decry that they could no longer "look their grandparents in the eye" or maintain friendships with others who voted contrary to their belief! One of us is married to a partner who votes for a different political party—in fact, we both belong to a generation where this is not uncommon. And yet, here were young people in their droves de-platforming grandma and de-friending anyone in their peer group who didn't vote for their preferred outcome! A very sorry state of affairs we would argue.

We cannot begin to impart how bizarre this looked from one generation to the next. It is small wonder people are unable to maintain friendships and keep family bonds together, when a political disagreement is enough to see the non-believers excommunicated permanently. The mind boggles as to how anyone with this fixed and rigid attitude could successfully keep a long-term marriage together, or tolerate children who horror of horrors, might grow up with a mind of their own. We could now add in many political disagreements across the world since Brexit—it seems to be a unanimous opinion among journalists and editors that people are becoming increasingly "polarised", backing themselves and others into a corner and shutting out any nuanced, alternative or different point of view to their own. Unfortunately, media, and its evil twin social media, then reinforce and validate these extreme positions by producing information that is so absurdly one-sided (be it on the left or right of politics) that no shades of grey or "other side of the story" is requested or offered. Instead, any opposing perspective or even gentle inquiry is immediately branded as some kind of "ist" or "phobic", and those who dare hold a different view are sentenced without trial to a hated out-group.

From a psychological point of view—herein lies the problem—even if we disagree most vehemently with a person's perspective, failure to at least attempt to understand why that person thinks that way removes the opportunity for a meaningful and constructive dialogue that might ultimately pave the way for mind-change, compromise or at the very least some empathy. It is possible to disagree very strongly with another's point of view, and yet have empathy for it. We might disagree strongly with another's decision to steal. But in listening to their rationale (even if we disagree with that as well) we can build understanding and empathise with the circumstances or background that led them to this point. We can still say hand on heart, we wouldn't have done the same in their situation, but we can see why they made that decision. This doesn't mean we agree with stealing, nor condone it, nor think they have a reasonable excuse. But opening your heart and mind to try to discern the motives of others will build your own Theory of Mind and broaden your perspectives. There is a lot of wisdom in the old saying: you have one mouth and two ears—use in proportion.

We hope that the points we are making do make sense. We also suggest that all parents should be uneasy and concerned with any signs that their children are withdrawing from the world, thinking only of themselves (always) and seeking out like-minded tribal bonds. Perspective-taking and empathy building has become yet another casualty in the Millennials and minus generations. Instead of working through difficult scenarios and complex problems in real life, with their peers, it's much easier to log onto social media and be fed a pack of lies by an algorithm designed to momentarily bolster an ego and a faux feeling of social inclusion. This also has an impact on how a young person views themselves and their place in the world; topics we explore in greater detail in Chap. 7. For now, however, we would like to provide you with other insights into how screens and screen time are impacting on the young people around us. The next chapter offers such an exploration.

Summary

Chapter 4 explored the concerning relationship between excessive screen time and neurodevelopmental outcomes in children and adolescents. Emerging research suggested that "Intensive Early Screen Exposure" correlates with autism-like behaviours, with studies showing that 1–2 hours of screen time at age one doubles the risk of ASD diagnosis by age three. The neurological mechanism for this appears linked to disrupted development of critical social skills, particularly Theory of Mind—the ability to understand others' perspectives. When screens displace real-world social interactions during sensitive developmental periods, children fail to build essential neural pathways for emotional recognition and social reciprocity. This parallels historical cases of severe social deprivation, like Genie Wiley, who demonstrated irreversible developmental deficits. The documented 17-fold increase in ASD diagnoses over 50 years, doubling in the last 20, coincides with widespread screen technology adoption. The research noted above suggests that these trends may contribute to increasing narcissism, declining empathy, and rising social polarisation observed in younger generations.

Bibliography and Further Reading

Baio et al. (2018). Prevalence of Autism Spectrum Disorder Among Children Aged 8 Years - Autism and Developmental Disabilities Monitoring Network, 11 Sites, United States, 2014. *Morbidity and Mortality Weekly Report – Surveillance Summaries*; Washington, D.C. 2018 Apr 27;67(6):1–23. https://doi.org/10.15585/mmwr.ss6706a1

Dadvand et al (2018). The association between lifelong greenspace exposure and 3-dimensional brain magnetic resonance imaging in Barcelona schoolchildren. *Environmental Health Perspectives*, 126(2). https://doi.org/10.1289/EHP1876

Dong, H.Y., Feng, J.Y, Wang, B., Shan, L. & Jia, F.Y. (2021) Screen Time and Autism: Current Situation and Risk Factors for Screen Time among Pre-School Children with ASD. *Frontiers in* Psychiatry, 12:675902. https://doi.org/10.3389/fpsyt.2021.675902

Fitzsimmons, C. (2023). Frances Haugen blew the whistle on Facebook two years ago. This is what happened next. The Sydney Morning Herald, October 9, 2023.

Giedd, J. (2001). *Frontline: Inside the teenage brain – An interview with Professor Jay Giedd.* Television documentary. Arlington Virginia: Public Broadcasting Service.

Harle, B. (2019) Intensive early screen exposure as a causal factor for symptoms of autistic spectrum disorder: The case for Virtual autism. *Trends in Neuroscience and Education*, 17, 100119. https://doi.org/10.1016/j.tine.2019.100119

Heffler K.F., Sienko D.M., Subedi K., McCann K.A., Bennett D. S. (2020) Association of early-life social and digital media experiences with development of autism spectrum disorder–like symptoms. *JAMA Pediatrics* 174(7):690–696. https://doi.org/10.1001/jamapediatrics.2020.0230

Hutton, J.S., Dudley, J., Horowitz-Kraus, T., DeWitt, T. & Holland, S.K. (2020). Associations between screen-based media use and brain white matter integrity in preschool-aged children. *JAMA Pediatrics*, 174(1), e193869. https://doi.org/10.1001/jamapediatrics.2019.3869.

Khan, A., Lee, E. Y., Rosenbaum, S., Khan, S. R., & Tremblay, M. S. (2021). Dose-dependent and joint associations between screen time, physical activity, and mental wellbeing in adolescents: an international observational study. *The Lancet. Child & Adolescent Health*, *5*(10), 729–738. https://doi.org/10.1016/S2352-4642(21)00200-5

Kushima et al., (2022). Association between screen time exposure in children at 1 year of age and autism spectrum disorder at 3 years of age The Japan Environment and Children's Study. JAMA Pediatrics, 176(4), 384–391. https://doi.org/10.1001/jamapediatrics.2021.5578

Sadeghi, S., Pouretemad, H.R., Khosrowabadi, R., Fathabadi, J. & Nikbakht, S. (2021). Parent–child interaction effects on autism symptoms and EEG relative power in young children with excessive screen-time, Early Child Development and Care, 191(6), 827–836. https://doi.org/10.1080/03004430.2019.1649256

Slobodin, O., Heffler, K.F. & Davidovitch, M. (2019). Screen media and autism spectrum disorder: A systematic literature review. *Journal of Developmental & Behavioral Pediatrics* 40(4), 303–311. https://doi.org/10.1097/DBP.0000000000000654

Uhls, Y.T., Michikyan, M., Morris, J., Garcia, D., Small, G. W., Zgourou, E., & Greenfield, P. M. (2014). Five days at outdoor education camp without screens improves preteen skills with nonverbal emotion cues. *Computers and Human Behavior, 39*, 387–392.

5

Lost in the Glow!

Attention is a limited resource, so pay attention to where you pay attention.
—Howard Rheingold

Abstract This chapter unpacks how modern screen technology affects human attention and cognitive development. It documents concerning cases of children exhibiting "virtual autism" due to excessive screen use, including behavioural problems when screens are removed. The information presented contrasts our evolutionary cognitive development—which thrived on natural environments and quiet reflection—with today's fragmented attention patterns driven by devices designed to manipulate our dopamine systems through irregular intermittent reinforcement. The chapter provides examples of research indicating that excessive screen time correlates with attention difficulties similar to ADHD, while exposure to natural environments can improve cognitive function. It also argues that constant digital distraction impairs critical developmental processes, including Theory of Mind, metacognition and deep-thinking abilities. Finally, the emphasis of the importance of modelling healthy screen habits and providing opportunities for children to engage with the

M. C. Nagel, R. Sharman, *Virtual Autism and Other Screen Disorders*, Palgrave Studies in Cyberpsychology, https://doi.org/10.1007/978-3-032-00803-9_5

natural world to support optimal cognitive and social development is set out as way forward for healthy overall development.

Keywords Attention • Dopamine • Attention Deficit Hyperactivity Disorder (ADHD) • Metacognition

Seeing Is Believing

Following the release of our first book tackling some of the topics here, Rachael received a phone call from a professional colleague and clinical psychologist at the coalface about her concerns in working with children displaying features of what would later become known as "virtual autism". The phone call in question came from a colleague who specialises in working with children and young people with a range of cognitive impairments. It is of note that this particular colleague is both highly qualified and experienced, and often sought out for a "second opinion" in highly complex cases.

Rachael's colleague began with "I haven't read your book yet, but I know what you're looking at, and I just wanted to discuss the following…" Said colleague had been contracted to provide additional testing and intervention for two primary-school aged boys. Both labelled as "Autism level 2" and both school refusers. The parents were at their wits end, having been unable to keep either child at school for more than a few days at a time across their combined schooling years.

After meeting with the parents, she asked to do something a little unorthodox: a home visit. To meet the boys in their own environment lest it lend clues as to their current predicament. Permission for the visit was granted and upon entering the home, she was first greeted with the sight of a seven-year-old boy who sat at a desk, earphones firmly in place, glued to a computer screen. What took her by surprise was that next to the computer screen was an I-pad, and it became rapidly apparent that the boy was "switching" between both devices as a constant stream of games played on each. If one game lagged, or became temporarily boring, he could switch immediately to the other on the other device. This back and forth allowed the boy to avoid being disconnected and un-entertained for even a matter of seconds. Relatedly, the younger brother was curled up on the couch, equally cut off from reality via headphones and immersed in an I-pad.

Upon further discussions with the parents, she ascertained that neither boy spent any discernible amount of time separated from their screens, which almost always accompanied them to dinner tables and anywhere they travelled. Just to add extra mortification to this situation, the parents acknowledged that when it came to bedtime, they drugged both boys to get them to sleep. They further stated that if the children awoke during the night, they would find them once again glued to their screens. And while home life was certainly a problem, attempts to get them to school were met with aggressive screaming, fighting and violence. Even at their children's early age and stages of development, their parents no longer had any capacity to manage them.

Anecdotes are often decried by critics but before you think this must be an extreme isolated case, a few short months later this very type of scenario made its way into mainstream news, as an increasingly common problem.[1] Turns out that hospital emergency departments, you know, those places meant to help people with heart attacks, car accidents, life and death scenarios, had increasingly become a repository of highly aggressive and out-of-control children who had their screen devices taken away. In the end, ER doctors, who were trained to save lives and generally have much more important things to be doing, were left pleading with parents to take an active role in parenting and remove their children's "digital cocaine" for good.

So, let's reflect, for a moment, on Rachael's colleague's "autistic" patient. Picture in your mind a young child straddled between two screens and switching between both and unable to tolerate even a few seconds at a time of non-entertainment or diversion. A worthy consideration would be what this is doing to this child's attentional development. To add some depth to this discussion let's allow our minds to wander back in time.

Evolutionary psychologists posit that the human ability to create fire gave rise to more than a convenient heating and cooking source. As we

[1] https://www.abc.net.au/news/2024-07-11/hospitalised-aggressive-children-urged-to-digital-detox/104056528

huddled together in our caves, able to transcend the night/ day cycle to remain awake and engaged past sundown, we began to find ways to amuse and entertain ourselves when the day's work was done. Indeed, that end-of-day reflection, simply sitting and staring into the fire, is legitimately thought to have given rise to one of our most extraordinary assets: our imagination.

The human capacity to work with, manipulate, and even invent abstract concepts 'in our heads' is unparalleled by any other species. Starting as early as six months of age, the human baby begins to demonstrate a cognitive ability psychologists refer to as 'object permanence'. Consider what happens after a ball rolls under a couch. An enthusiastic dog may scratch and whine for a while, but eventually will lose interest and wander off when distracted (think squirrel!). Human babies however, and with a few months maturation behind their cerebral belts, begin to understand that out of sight is not out of mind; they understand that the object they have lost still exists in space and time. Infants have even been shown to stare longer at apparent 'magic' tricks that suggest physical impermanence, suggesting they already understand this is not possible.

Now, fast forward about 12 years, when those magnificent frontal lobes explode in sophistication, and all of a sudden being able to mentally represent that ball under the couch transcends a capacity for understanding object permanence into being able to work with abstract concepts, algebra, even complex mathematical proofs—juggling all manner of information in our heads.

In earlier times, this extraordinary human ability to "play with things in our heads" translated to early artworks in caves, experimentation with different resources to invent solutions to practical problems (pottery, metals), storytelling, singing and dancing, the shared communication and transmission of ideas—all of which no doubt contributed to the continued development of ingenuity. Something further worth considering regarding our early ancestors. Without the constant distractions today's human beings encounter daily, and particularly in relation to screen devices, might some of our higher-order capacities been facilitated and developed by the time and space afforded to engage in the quiet reflection, meditation and processing of new information as our ancestors sat and stared quietly into the fire? After all, even Albert Einstein noted that "the monotony and solitude of a quiet life stimulates the creative mind".

Your Undivided Attention Please!

Have you ever taken some time to consider what you pay attention to and why? What holds your gaze, engages your thoughts, and when might your attention be captured elsewhere or start to drift? Or why you can be so engrossed in something that time passes exponentially without you even noticing.

Much more is now known about modern human attention capacity, its strengths, weaknesses and limitations. Many have probably heard of the seven plus or minus two capacity of our working memory or what is sometimes referred to as Miller's Law and named after the American psychologist, Dr George A Miller.[2] Miller's seminal work and paper on this topic in cognitive psychology is one of the most cited in psychology. Simply put, Miller's Law notes that most people can juggle between five and nine items in their head (shopping lists, phone numbers etc.) before they become overwhelmed. What is also known, but not as well understood, is that all our attentional faculties have limits—there are simply only so many things we can process at once. An Invisible Gorilla offers food for thought around this topic.

The reference to an Invisible Gorilla above is not an error but in fact the name of one of the most famous psychological experiments and subsequent book by Professors Christopher Chabris and Daniel Simons.[3] In their experiment, observers are presented with two teams of three or four individuals. One team is wearing white t-shirts while the other is dressed in black. While watching the teams, the participants are asked to count the number of ball passes made by one of the selected teams as they move around and pass the ball among their similarly clad team members. Not long after the experiment starts, another actor dressed in a gorilla suit then walks into the middle of the group, does a brief dance while beating its chest, and wanders off screen. This is where it gets interesting. After the teams stop passing the ball, the observers are asked to reveal how

[2] Miller (1956).

[3] Chabris and Simons (2010).

many passes were made. Those who get the number of passes correct rarely, if ever, noticed the gorilla unless previously told or cued to do so. They are so focused on completing the task of counting passes, they miss the glaringly obvious human masquerading as one of our primate cousins.

As unbelievable as this sounds, when replicated the experiment unfolds this way every time. It also confirms that there's only so much that human beings can focus on at once. Our attentional focus has limits, and if we've been given a task to do, we can easily overlook a distraction if it is unrelated to that task. We can also find ourselves in trouble if we try to pay attention to too many things at once; something the advent of ZOOM meetings has thrust upon many unwitting workers.

Many of you, especially since the COVID pandemic, have been afforded opportunities to work from home and as such this might sound familiar. You're in your home office involved in a staff meeting via ZOOM where someone is droning on about something you find difficult to give your undivided attention. You then check your diary to confirm when this meeting will end and any other business you will need to attend to that day or that week. Once you have made note of all that is in your diary you notice that a bird has landed in the branch outside your window or that your dog is suddenly making short work of one of your favourite slippers. After a moment of bird and/or dog watching you turn your attention back to the meeting only to hear that Phil is now offering a debrief of the most recent occupational health and safety meeting, which in your mind has no relevance to you or what you do. Your brain is crying out for something to help you stay alert, so you look for a dopamine hit from a game you downloaded on your phone or by doing some online shopping. Moments later, your surge of pleasure from hurling angry birds at pigs or purchasing the latest on trend fashion is then quickly replaced with panic as your boss calls out your name for your opinion on the topic at hand! So much for multi-tasking!!

People often misinterpret the phrase 'multi-tasking' and conflate it with attention in the belief that we can do numerous things simultaneously. This is true when it comes to walking and chewing gum or playing an instrument while singing but in terms of actively paying attention to something, your brain can only do one thing at a time. An important consideration in many of life circumstances such as trying to operate a phone while driving or playing games while in a staff meeting. There are limits to our attention!

As well as the growing understanding of the limitations of attention, we also know that it can be manipulated. It's no coincidence that some of our most highly paid psychiatrists and psychologists are employed by marketing companies and advertisers. Their job is to ensure they can attract and maintain customers' attention long enough for them to form a positive impression of whatever product they are trying to flog. Bonus points if they can convince them that they truly need a product that they almost certainly do not.

For those professionals who seek to gain and maintain your attention, the advent of the ubiquitous screen in your pocket has created a new focal point that can be commandeered by marketers to their full benefit. Their job is to ensure you leap to attention and check your phone the second you hear that 'ding'! Sounds familiar? The easiest way to do this is to invoke the training technique known as 'irregular intermittent reinforcement' and easily observable in gambling machines such as pokies or slots as they are known elsewhere.

We all like rewards but it turns out that there is something about our brains that prefers random rewards. Irregular intermittent reinforcement basically means to give rewards at random intervals without any predictable pattern. This in turn creates a sense of suspense and unpredictability that leads us to persist at something in the hope that we get a reward. If a reward is then randomly provided it offers a powerful reinforcement for continuing the behaviour. This particular way of delivering rewards excites you and lights up your "anticipatory dopamine" systems.

If you recall from Chap. 2, dopamine is a neurotransmitter or chemical messenger in the brain that creates feelings of pleasure and seeks rewards, which can drive you to repeat specific behaviours. Of interest here, and alluded to above, is that the unpredictability of receiving a reward increases anticipation and dopamine release or what is known as 'anticipatory' dopamine. Why is anticipatory dopamine so important? Consider the buzz you get when you smell bread breaking, or the crackling atmosphere in the stadium before a game begins, or how the heart flutters before the love of your life walks into a room. The experience of anticipation is almost always more exciting than finally engaging in the real thing. Let's face it … coffee never tastes as good as it smells.

Anticipatory dopamine is an incredibly powerful force as it drives us to 'do something' in order to access a reward. Even if we are disappointed time after time, all of a sudden, when we least expect it, bingo! We receive our prize. So, we leap to attention to answer the 'ding' on our phones because even though it's more likely to be a mundane text from our mum, friend, or work colleague—we are excited at the randomness and thoughts of that exciting person we're hoping to date, or a promising job offer we've been waiting on? The anticipation drives us to answer.

These same methods for engaging our anticipatory dopamine, with the help of technology, are used to tune us into the news, updates, information—most of the time it's mind-numbingly boring nonsense, but every now and then it's extraordinary and important news. These techniques are deliberately used to manipulate people into responding time and time again to the 'ding' that usually heralds nothing more than pointless and useless information, in the faint hope that just for once something interesting pops up on our screen. Of concern here also is what is that constant beck and call, scrolling and searching for something remotely interesting, taking us away from?

Australian cartoonist Michael Leunig found himself at the mercy of various social apologists and even accused of misogyny in 2019 when he dared to draw a cartoon depicting the truth of phone addiction for far too many parents and children.[4] His cartoon showed a mother so intent on her phone while wheeling the pram, that she hadn't noticed her baby had fallen out of it, and kept on walking, all the while fixated on her phone. Rather than inspire some self-reflection and community discussion about the misuse of technology and its broader impact in society, the personal abuse hurled at Leunig for daring to point out an ugly societal truth was well and truly in line with what happens to anyone who tries to take a substance away from an addict.

[4] https://www.abc.net.au/news/2019-11-01/leunig-mother-phone-cartoon-backlash-column/11663936

Even more ironically, his cartoon appeared shortly after a series of news reports from lifeguards and managers of council pools noting an increase in the rise of near-deaths and actual fatalities from children drowning while their parents sat by, glued to their phones. Some of these children actually died while their parents sat by the pool preoccupied with scrolling through their devices. So instead of Leunig's cartoon being a wake-up call, a conga line of handwringers supporting parents' 'right' to relax and enjoy uninterrupted 'me-time' looked to castigate his satirical call to arms; for some it even appeared that a dead child via negligence was a lesser crime than asking parents to disconnect from their phones.

We would be remiss if we failed to point out that this is not just happening in Australia. Type into Google 'drownings, parents on phone' to see an international sweep of just how widespread this problem has become. Individuals, young and old, are becoming increasingly addicted to, and dependent on, their smartphones for constant entertainment, distraction and attention. Very much to the detriment of their own young. And while adults may grapple with their screen use, Silicon Valley and its technology obsessed inhabitants are more focused on engaging younger generations.

Any drug-dealer or tobacco company executive knows, the earlier a dependency is formed, the harder it is to break later in life. Addiction has the capacity for creating lifelong consumers and a range of issues. The sordid history of the tobacco industry is not confined to hiding its research on addiction in the 1950s where it actively suppressed addiction research and spread disinformation to the public to conceal the harms caused by smoking. Current internal documents, and dating as far back as the 1970s, show that tobacco companies have long considered children and youth as targets as lifelong consumers of tobacco due to the addictive nature of its products.[5] Hook them early and company stocks stay healthy!

Addiction to screens is not too dissimilar and receives greater attention in the next chapter. In terms of attention, however, it is worth noting that the constant dinging and delivery of information titbits is also driving down a young person's capacity to concentrate for long periods of time or pay attention to where it is needed. Relatedly, the inability to become

[5] World Health Organisation (2024).

engrossed in a novel, or work through complicated hypotheses, ideas and philosophies in the context of a series of constant interruptions is resembling a form of artificial ADHD in young people. In other words, being lost in the glow of screens appears to be wiring developing brains towards favouring decreasing 'bits' of information over long, complex thought processes.

Fragmenting Attention

ADHD stands for 'attention deficit hyperactivity disorder'. Cognitively speaking it involves a very poor working memory combined with poor impulse control. So kiddies with ADHD can appear "naughty" as they fail to concentrate, listen, follow through on instructions and become easily distracted. Boys remain more vulnerable than girls at a diagnosis rate of 4:1, and ADHD increases in the context of biological insult to the brain before birth (twins, premature birth, certain genetic variations). ADHD is one of the "most genetic" of all psychological conditions, and unusually for a developmental disorder, it can be corroborated using MRI technologies looking into the brain. However, some recent environmental research has suggested the ADHD trajectory could be made better or worse via some surprisingly simple pathways.

Let's start by recognising demographic research showing lower rates of diagnosis in boys being raised in rural areas, and diagnostic rates decreasing the shorter the distance boys lived from a park.[6,7] Speaking of parks … in 2009, researchers found that children clinically diagnosed with ADHD could concentrate better after a 20-minute walk in the park![8] In this study children with ADHD completed a series of challenging puzzles to raise attentional fatigue before they walked through three different environments one week apart. One walk was through a vegetation-rich urban park while the other two were through the streets of a downtown area and an area clustered with houses respectively. After each walk, various aspects

[6] Donovan et al. (2019).

[7] McCormick (2017).

[8] Taylor and Kuo (2009).

of attention and executive functioning were also tested and walking through the park showed much better performance on those tests than walking in the other environments. In fact, walking through nature showed comparable results on tests of attention to other children who had taken the tests while medicated with methylphenidate or what is commonly known as Ritalin. The researchers concluded that doses of nature might serve as a safe, inexpensive, widely accessible non-medical tool for managing ADHD; being outside amongst mother nature may be better medicine than what is purchased at a pharmacy.

In a more recent study of more than 900,000 people published in 2019, researchers found that those who had access to a large amount of green space where they lived during childhood were significantly less likely to be at risk of developing a range of psychiatric disorders,[9] even after controlling for other known risk factors such as housing density, parental age and mental illness, and SES. In short, living within areas with a great deal of green spaces contributed to better mental health for those individuals across the lifespan. There have since been published several further studies that corroborate those findings.

Intriguingly brain imaging research has gone one step further, demonstrating that closeness to green space during childhood was positively associated with both white and grey matter volume in the prefrontal cortex, specifically regions associated with cognitive test scores of working memory and reduced inattentiveness.[10]

All of these examples and the growing body of research supporting or mirroring them give us pause to think. Might growing up "naturally" reduce or even eliminate symptoms of ADHD as the child's brain develops? Is climbing trees a better treatment option than medication? Should being in nature be a bigger priority than learning to code, playing online games, engaging in social media or regularly looking down while texting or 'influencing'.

We contend that those questions are both thought provoking and worthy of much discussion. Our contentions become even more compelling in the knowledge that over-exposure to screen time has now been shown

[9] Engemann et al. (2019).

[10] Dadvand et al. (2018).

to lead to white matter changes in the brain associated with language and attentional problems.[11] This leads to another thought, might screen environments be giving rise to attentional problems similar to ADHD? The evidence taken in its entirety certainly seems to suggest so, right down to neuronal development. Moreover, common sense itself should give rise to considering that if you are locked into a virtual world, how much time in the healthy confines of the natural world is being displaced.

Now let's go back now to our "normal" population. Assuming no background risk of attentional disorders is evident in the normal brain of a child, what might the knock-on effects be of our new ways of paying attention to the highway of information flooding in through our devices? We receive endless 'tweets', 'notifications' and 'headlines' all the time and more often than not they are tiny bits of information that act as clickbait but do little to inform us at any deep level. Their job is to make people react, and in that they are alarmingly successful. Have you ever considered how many people genuinely go behind the headline news to critically contemplate the information dispensed, and weigh up the source, their agenda, or even the logical consistency (or lack thereof) of the ideas being presented? Master manipulators have realised just how powerful a well-targeted message can be. Protests, even riots, can be easily triggered by a carefully crafted missile into a shallow attention span longing for a reason to react.

Remember our discussion of Theory of Mind from the previous chapter? This very skill, which is a significant deficiency in autism, also appears to be diminishing in younger cohorts. Considering the information presented above we posit the following question for your reflection. If someone has a diminished ability or completely lacks the attentional capacity to contemplate, process, abstractly reason and critically think about another person's perspective, what is that doing to their Theory of Mind? Trying to put yourself in someone else's shoes and get a sense of what they are thinking or how they are feeling is challenging, especially when the ability to pay attention to what they are saying or focus on their facial cues or body language is compromised. Moreover, because the brain is still maturing well into the third decade

[11] Hutton et al. (2020).

of life, children and adolescents who spend a great deal of time in a virtual world are distracted from the absolutely critical periods of developing any of the skills discussed above in the real world; being forever elsewhere is a recipe for all measures of cognitive, social and emotional deficits.

We'd like you to also consider the fact that thinking is effortful and actually 'improves' with age and practice. An important aspect of thinking is something called metacognition. Metacognition is about having an awareness of our thought processes or more simply being able to think about thinking or engage in deep reflection. Metacognitive abilities improve with age and experience. For example, we know that children perform disproportionately worse in metacognitive activities than adolescents and young to middle-aged adults while older adults show a decline with age.[12] Yes, it is an unfortunate reality that with ageing comes various measures of decline in our cognition and memory which can sadly be exacerbated by dementia or Alzheimer's disease. This should not be all that surprising. An infant's capacity to think about things beyond being hungry or uncomfortable will vastly improve with age and that infant's grandparent's older and well-worn brain may have to work very hard to remember where they put their eyeglasses.

As a bit of a metacognitive exercise, take a moment to reflect upon the more complex tasks your brain can undertake given the opportunity. Of course, it's easier to sit back and be a passive recipient of entertainment, and there's absolutely nothing wrong with giving your brain a rest at the end of a hard day. But can you recall the last time you really 'thought' about a topic? It didn't have to be some social issue de jour or some major event. Maybe you needed to consider what you're doing in your career, your relationship, as a parent, with your health. Or can you recall when you earnestly devoted some real thinking time to process, work through, gather information and develop a better understanding of your situation and your future goals? Entertaining these types of questions via reflection or thinking about your thinking is part of what it means to be human. Relatedly, another seriously important consideration is that of parents modelling the types of cognitive activities noted throughout this chapter in conjunction

[12] Filippi et al. (2020).

with responsible screen use behaviours to their children. Such modelling shows children and adolescents from day one that there is a time and place for screens, and a time and place to fully engage in reality.

Now, as imperfect parents, we appreciate this is easier said than done. One of us (Rachael) had the joy of managing a toddler during the pandemic and is happy to admit an over-reliance on screens during lockdown. However, a rather horrifying trend started to appear. Said toddler started to have massive tantrums when the screen was removed, and it came as no surprise that a lot of the sites he was visiting employed exactly the same nefarious techniques of intermittent reinforcement noted earlier, only this time hidden within kids' videos.

As time passed, weaning this young person off the screen proved futile and ultimately the cold turkey approach was employed—when the lockdown lifted, the toddler was informed his tablet had broken (parental code for 'it is actually hidden upstairs in the wardrobe'). About 72 hours of whinging and occasional tantrums ensued until the impact started to weaken. It was a couple of weeks before he really got back to normal playing outside and with his toys. But here's the thing, managing a three-year-old tantrum is a vastly different undertaking from wrangling with a strong six-foot male 15-year-old's beastly meltdown.

Left to fester, what we are seeing far too often are parents who have allowed this addiction/distraction to drift on for too long. They wheel in their 15-year-old, totally addicted to the latest video game, refusing to go to school, or engage in any social activity. Depression and anxiety are inevitable byproducts. Perhaps it's not too late to help this screenager and his exasperated parents, but it's exceedingly more difficult to remedy.

For mental health professionals and educators, desperate parents will often present this altered human asking them to 'fix their kid'. Please have another read of Chap. 1 and remind yourself that the human brain wires itself to the environment, context and social milieu in which it is immersed. If your child's brain has been allowed to simmer in a world of online 'unreality' with all the deliberate tricks of addiction used to keep it there—what skills and abilities have they forsaken and what are they left with now? Our experience as researchers tells us that a great deal of critical human capacities and abilities are being displaced via the addictively divine glow of screens. The chapters of this book are a reflection of that assertion and are supported by an ever-expanding array of research saying as much. However, even if you find some of the ideas we have presented thus far contentious, you can still personally engage with, or model to your children, activities that make for a better brain. By ensuring you seek opportunities to disengage from the constant distraction of screens, which invites shallow attention formation, you will be offering the opportunity to think, to dream, to process and reason with difficult concepts. Challenge that magnificent organ between your ears to its full capacity, instead of keeping it amused with pointless titbits scattered thought and superficial relationships. Concentrate, try to see something from another's perspective—we are all better people for cultivating these abilities. And just like our ancestors before us, allow some time and patience to contemplate so our clever brains can work to their potential, which remains vital to the development of understanding, imagination and ingenuity. Most importantly, let the young people around you see do this!

Summary

This chapter unpacked how modern screen technology affects human attention and cognitive development. It documented concerning cases of children exhibiting "virtual autism" due to excessive screen use, including behavioural problems when screens are removed. The information presented contrasted our evolutionary cognitive development—which thrived on natural environments and quiet reflection—with today's fragmented attention patterns driven by devices designed to manipulate our dopamine systems through irregular intermittent reinforcement. The chapter provided examples of research indicating that excessive screen time correlates with attention difficulties similar to ADHD, while exposure to natural environments can improve cognitive function. It also argued that constant digital distraction impairs critical developmental processes, including Theory of Mind, metacognition and deep-thinking abilities. Finally, the emphasis on the importance of modelling healthy screen habits and providing opportunities for children to engage with the natural world to support optimal cognitive and social development is set out as way forward for healthy overall development.

Bibliography and Further Reading

Chabris, C. & Simons, D. (2010). *The Invisible Gorilla: And Other Ways Our Intuitions Deceive Us*. Harmony.

Dadvand et al (2018). The association between lifelong greenspace exposure and 3-dimensional brain magnetic resonance imaging in Barcelona schoolchildren. *Environmental Health Perspectives*, 126(2). https://doi.org/10.1289/EHP1876

Donovan, G.H., Michael, Y.L., Gatziolis, D., Mannetje, A, & Douwes, J. (2019). Association between exposure to the natural environment, rurality, and attention-deficit hyperactivity disorder in children in New Zealand: A linkage study. *The Lancet: Planetary Health*, 3(5), E226–E234. https://doi.org/10.1016/S2542-5196(19)30070-1

Engemann, K., Pederson, C.B., Arge, L., Tsirogiannis, C., Mortenson, P.B. & Svenning, J.C. (2019). Residential green space in childhood is associated with lower risk of psychiatric disorders from adolescence into adulthood. *Proceedings of the National Academy of Sciences*, 116(11), 5188–5193. https://doi.org/10.1073/pnas.1807504116

Filippi, R., Ceccolini, A., Periche-Tomas, E. & Bright, P. (2020). Developmental trajectories of metacognitive processing and executive function from childhood to older age. *Quarterly Journal of Experimental Psychology*, 73(11), 1757–1773. https://doi.org/10.1177/1747021820931096

Hutton, J.S., Dudley, J., Horowitz-Kraus, T., DeWitt, T. & Holland, S.K. (2020). Associations between screen-based media use and brain white matter integrity in preschool-aged children. *JAMA Pediatrics*, 174(1), e193869. https://doi.org/10.1001/jamapediatrics.2019.3869.

McCormick, R. (2017). Does access to green space impact the mental well-being of children: A systematic review. *Journal of Pediatric Nursing*, 37, 3–7. https://doi.org/10.1016/j.pedn.2017.08.027

Miller, G.A. (1956). The magical number seven, plus or minus two: some limits on our capacity for processing information, *Psychological Review*, 63(2), 81–97. https://doi.org/10.1037/h0043158

Taylor, A.F. & Kuo, F.E. (2009). Children with attention deficits concentrate better after walk in the park. *Journal of Attention Disorders*, 12(5), 402–409. https://doi.org/10.1177/1087054708323000

World Health Organisation (2024). *Hooking the Next Generation: How the Tobacco Industry Captures Young Customers*. World Health Organisation, Geneva.

6

Social Media or Social Disease? Viruses of the Mind!

To become independent, find emotional support beyond the family, and find and keep a sexual partner, an adolescent must develop nuanced, sophisticated social skills. A lot of psychological changes happening in adolescents are therefore related to how we perceive, respond to, think about and interact with other people, For this reason, adolescence is known as a period of significant "social reorientation".
—Dr Lucy Foulkes (2021, p. 120)

Abstract This chapter focuses on interrogating how screen devices and social media platforms impact adolescent identity formation, with particular focus on teenage girls. As adolescents navigate the challenging physiological and psychological changes of puberty, the chapter posits that social media has created unprecedented avenues for identity exploration that often prove harmful. It also highlights how adolescent girls, already prone to negative emotions and body image concerns during puberty, now face additional pressures through constant social comparison with idealised online personas. This has contributed to alarming increases in mental health issues including anxiety, depression and self-harm behaviours. The chapter identifies concerning trends, including a

M. C. Nagel, R. Sharman, *Virtual Autism and Other Screen Disorders*, Palgrave Studies in Cyberpsychology, https://doi.org/10.1007/978-3-032-00803-9_6

dramatic rise in gender dysphoria among adolescent girls, suggesting social contagion facilitated by online communities as a contributor to such phenomenon. Through examining historical and contemporary examples of social contagion, the information presented in the chapter illustrates how social media has amplified the spread of harmful behaviours by allowing impressionable adolescents continuous access to damaging ideas and influences without appropriate guidance.

Keywords Identity • Puberty • Neuroticism • Social media • Social contagion • Gender dysphoria • Bandwagoning

Throughout this book we have introduced you to ideas and research suggesting that screen devices and their platforms are having an increasingly negative impact on the minds of the young people around us. Chapter 4 explored how time on screens may be altering the brains of children and adolescents alike in ways we are only beginning to understand. We specifically looked at a nascent but exploding phenomenon known as 'virtual autism' and how time on screens can be correlated to deficits in aspects of 'theory of mind'. Remember, Theory of Mind is our ability to put ourselves in someone else's shoes and consider different perspectives. The previous chapter took specific aim at what young people are looking at and how this impacts on their mental health. This chapter moves the discussion further and explores how tweens and teens might actually be losing themselves and having their identity shaped by people and events fed to them via algorithms in social media. This discussion begins by thinking about who we think we are!

Identity and the Self

Who are you? How do you see yourself? Are you the same person in public, in private, with friends, family or at work? Whilst it might seem on face value that consistency is a good thing, think again. Would you honestly admit some of your deepest feelings to a work colleague, friend, even partner? How about to yourself? How many secrets of the self do you hold?

Now you may be thinking that these types of questions are some form of philosophical navel gazing. But our sense of self and aspects of our identity impact on all aspects of our lives. For example, intimacy-building relies on the revelation of yourself, your real self, your beliefs, feelings, desires to another who accepts, values and maybe even reciprocates your thoughts. In the film *Avatar*, the Na'vi did not profess love for one another, but professed a simpler but more profound "I see you". "Seeing" into another person's innermost self is the basis for our strongest intimate partnerships.

Psychological researcher and Emeritus Professor Harry C Triandis pondered the difference between a 'Public' and 'Private' self that we all embody.[1] Most people can relate to keeping their real opinions or values to themselves while in public or in an unknown group of people. We lay off any tawdry jokes, un-PC opinions or bad language until we get to know those around us. Once we are confident that our sense of humour or manner of speaking won't be misunderstood, and will be appreciated, we start to reveal ourselves bit by bit in a socially acceptable manner. This dance of social acceptance occurs all the while engaging our emotion recognition radar to determine how our expressions are being received. It's only in our most intimate relationships with deep connections that we can truly be "ourself". This is the person we are in the wee small hours of the morning when we are losing sleep as we ponder life's issues.

Thinking of 'ourselves' is important with potentially far-reaching consequences. Consider the following quote from Amos Oz:

> The fanatics are the violent ones, the ones who want to change you by force. The ones who will force you to change. They love you. They love you dearly. They love you more than they love themselves. The fanatic has no private life. He or she is one hundred per cent public. No private life. The fanatic gives no value to his or her life. He is eager to sacrifice his life for the sake of a cause, whatever cause, because he doesn't think much of his life. His life is empty. No family, no relationship, no warmth, no human touch to his life. One hundred per cent public.[2]

---

[1] Triandis (1989).

[2] Oz (2001).

Oz, (now deceased) grew up in war-torn Jerusalem and developed a profound insight into where extremist thinking leads. Interestingly he may well have prophesised the impact of increased polarisation and the loss of your true or "private" self in today's social media environment. Oz suggests that terrorists and other extremists lack a "private" self. This is an interesting way of framing extremist behaviour. Your private self is the part of you used for quiet reflection, learning and mind-change. This raises some important questions in the context of the propositions made in this book.

Remember the human brain is not fully developed and mature until we reach our mid to late twenties. For children, tweens and teens this means that their immature minds are potentially exposed to information they may not be able to process with any degree of nuance or sophisticated thinking. So, the move from childhood to adulthood is not always smooth, to say the least!

How many of you, given the chance, would be happy to relive your adolescent years. Would you be interested in reliving growth spurts with any measure of associated aches and pains, troubled skin conditions, menstruation, and many other physiological changes which are just the tip of the hormonal iceberg? How about having to, once again, venture through sensation-seeking and risk-taking behaviours coupled with fluctuations in moods, attitudes and behaviours as you try to distance yourself from your childhood and nurture independence away from your parents? Adolescence is challenging, complex and for some, a time of great anxiety and stress. It is also a time when young people are trying to find out who they are and where they fit in the world. During adolescence, young people are inventing their personas, and speaking themselves into existence where identity formation is a crucial component of this maturational journey.

Identity formation during adolescence has a long research history and many who work in this area often base their work on that of Erik Erikson. Erikson, a psychologist and psychoanalyst, developed his eight-stage theory of 'psychosocial development' in the 1950s. In his framework he framed adolescence as the time from 11 to 19 years of age and labelled it as a period of 'Identity versus Role Confusion'.[3] An important aspect of his theory is the notion that the shaping of one's identity is influenced by social dynamics with peers and mentors playing a significant role in the shaping of that identity.[4] It is also noteworthy that identity formation itself can only begin in adolescence because it requires cognitive capacities that are becoming available at that time. The immature brain of a child is not equipped to think about the shaping of their identity and instead are content acting like the family pet or 'being Batman' or any other fictitious character. Young children vacillate between many personas and identities simply because they are not cognitively sophisticated enough to do otherwise.

Many researchers have built on Erikson's work and it is now widely accepted that identity formation, through personal exploration and experimentation is a core developmental task through adolescence and into early adulthood. If this all sounds a bit technical think back to your times as an adolescent. What group or tribe did you attach yourself to? Were you a 'jock' or a 'headbanger'? Were you labelled a 'nerd', a 'geek', an 'emo' or a 'goth'? Every generation sees adolescents create labels and identities in response to working out who they are within the social and cultural milieu of the times. If your own memories elude you then watch the movies *Grease* or any of the *Twilight* films. Those films focus on high school students trying to work out who they are and who they are meant to be. Danny Zuko (John Travolta) evolves from being a 'T-Bird' to a jock so he could have a relationship with Sandy Olsson (Olivia Newton John). Bella Swan (Kristen Stewart) has feelings for the vampire Edward (Robert Pattison) and Jacob, a modern-day werewolf played by Taylor Lautner. Those movies were not simply about being part of a 'clique'. Instead, they provide examples of adolescents working out who they are and their place in the world. Unfortunately, they don't always depict what happens when, and how, things can go wrong.

As noted above, the shaping of one's identity is a core developmental task during adolescence. Because of this we know that those who struggle to forge a healthy sense of self are often prone to anxiety, depression and

[3] Erikson (1950, 1959).

[4] Erikson (1968).

a range of negative outcomes. Erikson, himself, argued that the inability to form a stable identity often leads to role confusion which in turn can manifest into anything from delinquency to psychotic episodes.[5] Indeed contemporary researchers argue that a majority of personality disorders are associated with an unstable identity or sense of self.[6] For us, a significant area of concern is to what extent social media is having a negative impact on identity formation during childhood and adolescence. What, for example, happens to someone who raises themselves and "develops" their opinions of themself and shapes their identity beyond the confines of close family and friends and via screen devices? At the time of writing, a glaringly obvious group of adolescents, namely adolescent girls, provides much food for thought.

Puberty Sucks! Especially for Girls!

Earlier we offered some insights into the developing brain during adolescence. We'd like to extend that conversation a bit further here as a framework for our meanderings about identity formation in girls.

If you recall, when children enter puberty, the brain begins a journey of reconstruction and fine-tuning. Although it might seem axiomatic to state, so too does the body and mind. Let's talk about these changes with broad brush strokes by noting from the outset that puberty is a very difficult time for girls. Comparatively speaking, puberty presents far greater challenges to girls and much more upheaval in terms of emotion and identity than what occurs for boys. There are a range of factors that likely contribute to this beyond the scope and intent of this chapter. Nonetheless, the research across many disciplines tells us that puberty is very problematic for girls. From cultural norms and expectations to bodily and physiological changes, puberty seems to present far more challenges and potential negative outcomes for girls.

One of the first challenges we can see has to do with how adolescents feel about themselves and the world. Prior to the onset of puberty boys

[5] Erikson (1950).

[6] Klimstra and van Doeselaar (2017); see also Kernberg and Caligor (2005).

and girls roughly experience similar levels of neuroticism or what you might simply call negative emotions. When children enter puberty, levels of neuroticism escalate in girls and this trend extends across the lifetime; it is well documented that females are far more likely to experience negative emotions such as anxiety, anger or depression than males. Relatedly, at a time when relationships and the desire to become an adult become increasingly important for girls so too does increasing hypersensitivity to negative emotions.

At the risk of stating the obvious, feeling bad is not good! The better we feel about ourselves and life in general, the better we are able to function, meet the challenges of each day and perform in most aspects of life. Neuroticism is the opposite of emotional stability and the tendency for experiencing negative feelings can lead to rather destructive outcomes, both physically and psychologically. For girls, much of their negative feelings focus on their bodies and their inner perceptions of how they look.

Body image is an important aspect of adolescent development for both boys and girls but is far more problematic for girls. As boys relish in newfound muscle mass, facial hair and deeper voices, girls are often embarrassed by their first period, curvier hips and developing breasts. Part of this problem is cultural but also can be found in the reality that girls enter puberty much sooner than boys and as such are often having many uncomfortable encounters with their immature male counterparts. For many girls, their bodies and the related changes to those bodies lead to a preoccupation with how they look and/or how they think they should look. This is particularly troublesome when linked with negative emotions.

When girls are inundated with negative emotions they tend to ruminate and engage in internalising thoughts and behaviours. Those thoughts and behaviours can be overwhelming when changes to the body are occurring and regularly result in adolescent girls spending a great deal of time in front of mirrors examining themselves. This is a bad scenario given that a preoccupation with appearance, especially perceived flaws or defects not observable to others, can result in a range of problematic outcomes. Couple this with the rampant use of technology and a need to take 'selfies', be 'liked' and garnish attention on social media and we see many girls investing in unrealistic ideals about beauty and how they should look and feel as they are forming their emerging identities.

Just to recap and before we look deeper at the pernicious nature of social media … puberty is very difficult for adolescent girls and negative emotions are commonplace at a time when body image is an important component of an emerging identity. Historically, such challenges, at the intersection of cultural notions of beauty, have resulted in many girls being dissatisfied with how they look. Such dissatisfaction has led to an array of anxiety-related disorders including, but not limited to, low self-esteem, depression, eating disorders, appearance rumination, cutting or self-mutilation, and body dysmorphic disorder. We would also contend, and increasing evidence supports us, that screens and social media have exacerbated those issues and have played a role in an explosive number of girls now claiming to be transgender.

Looking for Help in the Social-Media Vacuum

There is an age difference between us (the authors), but both of us have witnessed, in our lifetimes, adolescent girls struggling with their bodies and identities. Such struggles have, on occasion, and in our experience, manifested as eating disorders and as various degrees of bodily mutilation, cutting or self-harm. And don't get us wrong, these things still exist and doctors and mental health practitioners are still having to help and support young girls who self-harm in many ways. However, and as discussed in chapter three, somewhere around 2010, adolescents started using social media in ever expanding and pervasive ways. This included measuring and comparing their looks and lives with people online resulting in an exponential growth of anxious youth with severe mental health problems. This is true of both boys and girls but there appears to be a larger and more consistent relationship between girls, social media and increasing mental health issues. This could be due to the fact that while boys and girls started spending more time online since 2010, they spent that time differently. Boys were watching YouTube videos and playing multiplayer video games. For boys, challenges around screen devices focused on time and addiction to video games. Girls, on the other hand, were, and are, spending time on visual platforms where they compare themselves to others, desire to be 'liked' or seek guidance in all things they do or feel.

Consider the protagonist from *Gone with the Wind*, Scarlett O'Hara who was famed for having the smallest waist in three counties. Whilst girls and young women have always competed for attention on the basis of body shape, 200 hundred years ago how many competitors could they reasonably have? A few dozen in their age range, a hundred at most? Fast forward to today, and girls are comparing themselves with thousands upon thousands of air-brushed images that bear little relationship to reality. This in turn creates a false sense of normality and heightens the perceived flaws of each ruminating girl as she flicks through Instagram or similar.

Girls use social media to view the lives of others and often compare themselves to what they see online. Adolescent girls who are struggling with puberty will use social media to curate a false life, look to find some way to 'fix' themselves or their lives, ruminate over their negative emotions and/or find comfort in the online arms of others, who purportedly share similar thoughts, experiences and have their best interests at heart. For some young girls that has led to a strong desire for cosmetic surgery while for others it has meant disowning not only their true identities but also their bodies.

It is with a degree of trepidation that we discuss notions of gender identity and gender dysphoria. Since 2015 or so, this topic has become increasingly radioactive in the cultural zeitgeist. But at a time when girls are increasingly seeking out ways to change how they look and feel and finding support and pathways for doing so on social media we think it prudent to have this conversation.

Let's start by acknowledging that many generations of girls have looked to shape their identity by aspiring to look like someone popular or famous. Many girls have also struggled with pubescence and subsequent changes to their body. However, whereas previous generations found guidance, advice and support from family members or close friends during adolescence, today's girls are on social media curating false identities, ruminating with others about their 'sad' existence and/or seeking advice on why they don't like their bodies. This capacity for ruminating over negative emotions and expressing self-doubt about one's identity now extends beyond the home in a virtual world of 24/7 outside influence and 'influencers'. The results of this are only beginning to be understood but one area that stands out is the number of girls who are struggling with their gender identity.

A myriad of reports and studies show a massive increase in the number of adolescents, mostly girls, with some measure of discomfort with their biological sex and by association gender identity. This has manifested in an explosion of girls asserting that they are 'non-binary' or 'trans'. There is a reason we focus on girls here. Interestingly there are biological hypotheses and increasingly well-supported research that pinpoint the biological processes that may result in a chromosomal male (i.e., has a Y chromosome) feeling more in line psychologically with his female counterparts. It is beyond the scope of this book to delve into these, suffice to say in-utero hormonal impacts on the developing brain appear to be the main contender for giving rise to males "feeling" more female.[7]

However, whilst in-utero hormones also come under the spotlight for chromosomal females (do not have a Y chromosome) "feeling" male, this only accounts for a very tiny proportion and typically those with known androgen differences e.g., CAH. So where have all these other females, recently and rather suddenly feeling male, come from? The explosion in numbers is profound and extraordinary and while a recent review concluded the rapid rise in gender dysphoria for chromosomal females is currently for reasons unknown, it also noted the likelihood of social media as a major contributing factor.[8]

Some estimates suggest a four thousand percent increase of individuals claiming to be transgender from 2016 to 2023 across many countries but most notably the United States, Canada, the United Kingdom, New Zealand and Australia.[9] It is not unreasonable to suggest that there is an alternative hypothesis not nested in biology for this exponential rise in numbers. We would contend that there is possibly some form of peer or social contagion via social media at play here. Historically, gender

[7] Nguyen et al. (2019).

[8] Graham (2023).

[9] Grossman (2023).

dysphoria, or what was previously referred to in the clinical literature as gender identity disorder, occurred around the age that gender identity is formed (roughly four years) and afflicted a very small section of the population; mostly boys.

The research literature on the harms associated with smartphones and social media is compelling. Aspects of positive self-esteem, self-concept and self-confidence have plummeted in adolescents while anorexia, cutting, self-harm and suicide have all spiked dramatically since the arrival of the smartphone and social media.[10] It should not be any surprise that notions of identity, and in particular gender identity, during the vulnerable time of adolescence, have also been negatively impacted by social media. Adolescent girls, unhappy with the turmoil of puberty and their changing bodies, have turned to find help via social media.

If there are social media forces at play here (rather than biological) it is perhaps then of no surprise that it is during puberty that the transgender phenomenon flourishes amongst females. If, as activists would have you believe, the rise in transgenderism is a product of greater cultural acceptance, then where are the formerly closeted adults now proclaiming to be 'trans'? Rather, it appears to be that today's adolescent girls, unhappy with their bodies, have potentially fallen into a social media trap that fosters ruminating about issues beyond those related to food and cutting.

Today's adolescent girls turn to social media looking for quick fixes and often find advice from strangers and advocates who have their own self-interests, agendas and potential psychological issues. Make no mistake, social media is not a place where you can always rely on great expertise and sage advice and instead is a place parents need to monitor. It is somewhat of a paradox that many of today's parents are nervous or anxious about letting their children go out into the 'real' world on their own lest they be injured or abducted but do not give a second thought to the virtual world their children spend much of their time in; a world that is increasingly acknowledged as a place where predators and many nefarious individuals hide amongst their prey.

That last sentence may seem hyperbolic, but the evidence suggests otherwise. Whereas schools, playgrounds, and churches have historically

[10] Twenge (2017).

provided access to vulnerable children and adolescents, harming or abducting a young person was very difficult and very rare despite what news reports might have you think. Social media, on the other hand, is a space where it is far easier to hide one's identity and predatory inclinations. For example, in 2014, a ten-year-old girl had been groomed and targeted by at least 16 men on the iPad her parents had provided to her to help with her homework.[11] That was a decade ago and the technology and its associated platforms have advanced in use of ease and opportunity. At the time of writing such online predatory events have become, worryingly, all too common.

Social media is also a platform for enticement and where children and adolescents are lured to join online communities where life is promised to be prosperous, abundant and better.[12] For adolescent girls struggling with puberty, their body image and identity, social media becomes a place for co-rumination with others who feel terrible. It is also a space where 'influencers' lurk in the virtual shadows ever watchful for someone to 'help'. In previous decades it was the "thinspiration" anorexia/eating disorder proponents encouraging young girls to remain, young, in their body shape (i.e., retain a pre-pubescent shape). In the realm of gender dysphoria, promotion of trans is something to celebrate with the suggestion that those unhappy about puberty and body image may be in the wrong body altogether.[13] Perhaps this goes some way to explain the extraordinary increase in those who say they have been born in the wrong bodies? The desire to 'transition' might be called the latest 'fad' for the angst of growing up an adolescent female given the available statistics as there appears to be a form of contagion spreading among teenage girls who suddenly believe themselves to be boys.

We would also like to point out the clear difference here between those who, and with emphasis, make identity-affirming decisions as ***adults*** as opposed to children and adolescents who are at best, questionably capable of making such life altering decisions. Indeed, in Australia the age of 16 years is considered reasonable in terms of giving "informed consent"

[11] Linning (2014).

[12] Louie (2017).

[13] Shrier 2020.

for medical procedures (and entering a sexual relationship for that matter), with the usual caveats regarding intellectual or mental impairments. We couple our contention that social media has also created a perfect storm for 'bandwagoning ', and for social contagions to take hold of the lives of young people in a variety of realms. In this decade it just happens to be gender dysphoria that is all the rage. No doubt next decade we will look to a new replacement.

Social Media and the Spread of Anxiety and Mind Viruses

The preceding section explored the recent phenomenon of girls who suddenly believe themselves to be boys or devoid of biological sex altogether. We contend that this is another manifestation of the struggles girls face when they begin puberty and find discomfort in themselves as they try to work out who and what they are in terms of their identity. At this juncture we would also like to suggest that there are other things at play. Let's start with 'bandwagoning '.

The term 'bandwagoning ' is derived from the phenomenon in human behavioural science known as the 'bandwagon effect'. The bandwagon effect is a cognitive bias where people either believe that an idea or belief is true because many others believe it or have adopted it or where individuals favour a popular trend merely because it is popular.[14] In more colloquial parlance, we might often accuse someone of 'joining the bandwagon' when they switch their sporting allegiances, fashion sensibilities or political persuasions … everyone loves a winner or to 'be on trend'.

In the context of this chapter, it is our contention that social media offers a widespread and pervasive platform for bandwagoning. Whereas previous generation's access to cultural, social and populist trends was limited to their immediate environments, today's young people have unfettered 24/7 access to just about anything and/or anyone. For adolescent girls this might mean jumping onto the latest fad that may not be particularly positive or healthy. Eating disorders, self-harm and gender

[14] Sullivan (2009).

dysphoria provide avenues to jump on the bandwagon to compete for attention or find solidarity with other girls online. An anecdote helps to illustrate this.

In 2014 Michael gave a presentation on the developing adolescent brain to the parents of his son's high school in Brisbane. After the presentation he was approached by an ER doctor from one of Brisbane's largest hospitals who shared with him a phenomenon she was seeing in her practice as an attending ER physician. This doctor had been noticing something rather odd happening in the ER on a regular basis involving groups of teenage girls who had been making repeated visits to the ER due to self-harm—they were cutting themselves. The self-harm wasn't what was odd as there had been a long history of girls arriving in the ER with cutting injuries over the years. What caught the doctor's attention was that there were groups of girls who were arriving in the ER at the same time and on a regular basis. It turned out that they developed a pattern of ruminating about their 'terrible' lives collectively on social media, and then proceeded to cut themselves at the same time online so they could meet in the ER and ruminate in person. This group started out with three girls, but overtime others jumped on the cutting bandwagon for attention and not to be left out. It was only when groups grew in size and had their group angst and anger sessions more openly in the ER did the doctor and parents become suspicious. Such events, by their nature, do not happen in isolation and can also be linked to social contagions.

Monkey See, Monkey Do!

Human beings like to be part of a crowd. We are indeed social beings and the need to connect with others is in our evolutionary DNA. So much so that we often mirror the facial expressions and actions of those around us on a regular basis. Next time you are sitting across from someone having a chat do a little experiment. Make a conscious effort to shift your body language on a regular basis and watch the person you are engaged with…have a stretch of some sort, cross your arms, touch your face or hair, cross your legs, slouch back in your chair or the classic, simply yawn. As you do these things you may be surprised to see a great deal of mimicry going on by the person across from you. Your movements and mannerisms have become contagious.

We mimic the facial expressions of others, their vocal utterances, their movements and many other aspects of behaviour without realising it. So powerful is the innate desire to mimic, it appears that human beings can even pass their emotional states to another person. The Germans have captured the essence of this beautifully in one word 'Einfühlung'—to feel one's way into another person's experience. Sometimes feeling one's way into another person's experience goes beyond simple facial cues and individual behaviours. Sometimes individual experiences become part of a collective social contagion.

Social contagion occurs when information such as attitudes, emotions or behaviours are rapidly spread from one individual to others without rational thought and reason. Many times these can be harmless when people follow fads or trends. However, there are plenty of examples of modern social contagions causing harm which we will explore shortly.[15] Prior to looking at contemporary examples of harmful social contagions and connections to social media, it is important to note that social contagions are not new concepts and have a long history.

In 1774, Johann Wolfgang von Goethe's book 'The Sorrows of Young Werther' provided the catalyst to a now infamous social contagion. In this novel, Werther, a young man caught up in a love triangle eventually kills himself. As the book's popularity grew across Europe, a wave of young men ended their lives dressed in the same clothing as von Goethe's description of Werther. There are reports that some even had copies of the novel beside them with the book opened to pages of the suicide scene.[16] Some readers shot themselves with the same kind of pistol Werther used in the novel. In 1974, sociologist and suicide researcher, Dr David Phillips coined the term "The Werther Effect" to refer to the phenomenon of copycat suicides.[17] The research done by Phillips resulted in

[15] The seminal work of Hatfield et al. (1994) provides a cogent and detailed exploration of the phenomenon of emotional contagion.

[16] Jack (2014).

[17] Phillips (1974).

recommendations that stories about suicide should never be placed on the front page of newspapers.

Flash forward to present day where newspapers are not nearly as popular but where anyone of any age can access information online. Copycat suicides are seen in local clusters from time to time and presented as a product of social contagion. Henry M Gunn High School, in Palo Alto, California, the birthplace of Silicon Valley and the home of many wealthy families has experienced the 'Werther Effect' on more than one occasion. From 2009 to 2010, five students or recent graduates from Gunn High School committed suicide by standing in front of an oncoming train. Later, from October 2014 to March 2015, four more Palo Alto Unified School District students took their own lives. Most recently in February of 2024, a 16-year-old girl committed suicide also by standing in the path of a California train.

The factors that contributed to the deaths of so many young people in an affluential part of California are still debated, contested and beyond the scope of this book. What is not in doubt is that the tragic deaths noted above provided evidence that social contagions do exist; ten young lives lost by standing in front of an oncoming train is no coincidence. They are part of a recognised psychological and sociological phenomenon we refer to as a social contagion as is the capacity for such contagions to fester in the minds of young people via social media. Young people do not only follow fads and trends but will also engage in unhealthy and harmful behaviour as a byproduct of social contagion. Eating disorders, identity disorders, cutting behaviours and sadly suicide as described above are prime examples of the harmful effects of social contagion in the field of mental health.[18] And at a time when children and teens can mimic one another via social media and other online platforms 24/7, is it any wonder we are witnessing rising rates of mental health problems since 2010. Eric Hoffer, an American philosopher and recipient of the Presidential Medal of Freedom in 1993 noted that 'when people are free to do as they please, they usually imitate each other'.[19] They may also imitate others our of a fear of not being part of a group. Fear of missing

[18] Riggio and Riggio (2023).

[19] Hoffer (1955).

out (FOMO) is a particularly interesting extension of social contagion. FOMO on social media for teens and young adults tends to manifest as being a factor in motivating young people to be the first on the 'bandwagon'. They enthusiastically leap onto someone else's idea, platform or agenda to align themselves with others as quickly as possible. Such actions allow individuals to inherit some 'borrowed power' from the original source to propel them into some form of a leadership position. Moreover, teens will literally fall over themselves to become quickly aligned with whatever idea, movement or position that is likely to lead to popularity. What they actually think about the issue is largely irrelevant. This is where our final psychological concept of interest kicks in called Behavioural Activation Theory. This theory suggests that it is in fact behaviour that dictates belief, not the other way around. Perhaps it is helpful to think of Behavioural Activation Theory this way: when the average human engages in a behaviour, especially one that comes at cost to them, they must justify that act to themselves. Imagine 15-year-old Sally has posted a meme in favour of a political party. Sally is actually ambivalent about that party, but she is re-posting from an influential instagrammer, and Sally has been feeling a bit deflated lately, with not a lot of friends and not a lot of attention, so she's in the mood to boost her social standing via some borrowed power. So she gets in quick to forward the meme. It turns out Sally hits the social jackpot! All of a sudden she is being showered with likes. Everyone loves her! Her dopamine runneth over. She feels included, important, and even a bit clever for being one of the first groupies, if not the original source. But what does Sally actually stand for? Initially she stood for popularity, a bit of affiliation and an ego boost. Most of the Sallys of the world (and there are a lot of them) don't even know the ins and outs of the idea they support. They've spent zero time engaging in anything remotely close to critical analysis, and haven't bothered to think through the issues. They just wanted to be loved. When a difficult person comes along and asks a hard question about the substance of their beliefs they can't actually answer. Their inability to give a coherent answer lies in the fact that the basis of their behaviour wasn't driven by any actual belief. Instead, Sally was driven to improve her popularity first and mould her beliefs second. In the end, how is she likely to respond when her beliefs are questioned? She will likely have no idea of substance in this situation, and instead be very upset if it appears that her newfound popularity might be threatened. Now that's not to say people always re-post or support causes for the above reasons. Clearly there are true believers out there who have thought long and hard about their positions. In fact, you can employ a pretty easy tactic to find out who is the leader and who is the follower in these scenarios. Ask a question. Ask them to explain their rationale. And then watch their response. Are they able to articulate an argument for their position? An idea, even a thought? Remember what we previously discussed: In this type of situation, people who are frauds react by 'playing the man instead of the ball'. Instead of engaging in reasoned and interesting thoughtful discourse about the issue, they react instinctively and angrily (as anyone does when they feel threatened) and they shoot the messenger. In situations similar to Sally's, their primary concerns is if they are found out—because their 'beliefs' are entirely vacuous and they fear being revealed as an imposter. Add in a bit of faux outrage, and their insistence they are horribly offended and congratulations—they have now become an official cry-bully. Shooting the messenger who asked the valid question is achieved by tarring them with any kind unpleasant label, and calls for cancellation. That is the easiest and laziest way to ensure the fragile platform of ideas is never uncovered. Such approaches and tactics are now ubiquitous across social media platforms. There's rarely an original idea or critical thought, however, such online environments are awash with bandwagoning, passive-aggressive gaslighting and concerted mobbing by cry-bullies. In the end, previous generations may have considered imitation a form of flattery, but in a world of 24/7 access to social media, imitation may actually be harmful or deadly form of flattery.

Summary

Chapter 6 focused on interrogating how screen devices and social media platforms impact adolescent identity formation, with particular focus on teenage girls. As adolescents navigate the challenging physiological and psychological changes of puberty, the chapter posited that social media has created unprecedented avenues for identity exploration that often prove harmful. It also highlighted how adolescent girls, already prone to negative emotions and body image concerns during puberty, now face additional pressures through constant social comparison with idealised online personas. This has contributed to alarming increases in mental health issues including anxiety, depression and self-harm behaviours. The chapter identified concerning trends, including a dramatic rise in gender dysphoria among adolescent girls, suggesting social contagion facilitated by online communities as a contributor to such phenomenon. Through examining historical and contemporary examples of social contagion, the information presented above illustrated how social media has amplified the spread of harmful behaviours by allowing impressionable adolescents continuous access to damaging ideas and influences without appropriate guidance.

Bibliography and Further Reading

Erikson, E.H. (1950). *Childhood and Society*. Norton.

Erikson, E.H. (1959). Identity and the life cycle. *Psychological Issues*, 1, 1–171.

Erikson, E.H. (1968). *Identity, Youth and Crisis*. Norton.

Graham, P. (2023). Transgender children and young people: How the evidence can point a way forward. *BJPsyche Bulletin*, 47(2), 98–104. https://doi.org/10.1192/bjb.2022.3

Grossman, M. (2023). *Lost in Trans Nation: A Child Psychiatrists Guide Out of the Madness*. Skyhorse Publishing.

Hatfield, E., Cacioppo, J.T. & Rapson, R.L. (1994). *Emotional Contagion: Studies in Emotions & Social Interaction*. Cambridge University Press.

Hoffer, E. (1955). *The Passionate State of Mind, and Other Aphorisms*. Harper.

Jack, B. (2014). Goethe's *Werther* and its effects. *The Lancet Psychiatry*, 1(1), 18–19. https://doi.org/10.1016/S2215-0366(14)70229-9

Kernberg, O.F., & Caligor, E. (2005). A psychoanalytic theory of personality disorders. In M.F. Lenzenweger, & J. Clarkin (Eds.), *Major Theories of Personality Disorders* (2nd ed.). The Guilford Press.

Klimstra, T. & van Doeselaar, L. (2017). Identity formation in adolescence and young adulthood. In j. Specht (Ed.), *Personality Development Across the Lifespan*, Chapter 18, pp. 293–308. Academic Press. *Obesity Reviews*, 22(9), e13263. https://doi.org/10.1111/0br.13263

Linning, S. (2014). Is your child's new iPad a magnet for paedophiles? Ten-year-old girl groomed through tablet by perverts despite her parents taking 'all sensible safety measures', UK Daily Mail, 27th December. Available at https://www.dailymail.co.uk/news/article-2888300/Is-child-s-new-iPad-magnet-paedophiles-Ten-year-old-girl-groomed-tablet-perverts-despite-parents-taking-sensible-safety-measures.html (Accessed 1st May, 2024).

Louie, D.W. (2017). Social media and the sexual exploitation of Indigenous girls. *Girlhood Studies*, 10(2), 97–113. https://doi.org/10.3167/ghs.2017.100208

Nguyen, H.B., Loughead, J., Lipner, E., Hantsoo, L., Kornfield, S.L. & Epperson, C.N. (2019). What has sex got to do with it? The role of hormones in the transgender brain. *Neuropsychopharmacology*, 44(1), 22–37. https://doi.org/10.1038/s41386-018-0140-7

Oz, A. (2001). Big Ideas ABC Television. https://www.abc.net.au/radionational/programs/archived/radioeye/how-to-cure-a-fanatic%2D%2D-amos-oz/3475244#transcript

Phillips, D.P. (1974). The influence of suggestion on suicide: Substantive and theoretical implications of the Werther Effect. *American Sociological Review*, 39(3), 340–354. https://doi.org/10.2307/2094294

Riggio, R.E. & Riggio, C.R. (2023). Social Contagion in H.S. Friedman & C.H. Markey (Eds.), *Encyclopedia of Mental Health – 3rd Edition* (Vol 3, pp. 270–273). Elsevier. https://doi.org/10.1016/B978-0-323-91497-0.00192-2

Sullivan, L.E. (2009). *The SAGE Glossary of the Social and Behavioral Sciences.* SAGE Publications Inc.

Triandis, H.C. (1989). The self and social behaviour in differing cultural contexts. Psychological Review, 96(3), 506–520. https://doi.org/10.1037/0033-295X.96.3.506

Twenge, J.M. (2017). *iGen: Why Today's Super-Connected Kids Are Growing Up Less Rebellious, More Tolerant, Less Happy – and Completely Unprepared for Adulthood.* Atria Books.

7

Unwanted Influence: Cyberbullying, Violence and the Radicalised Mind!

...parasitic pathogens of the human mind ... these are composed of thought patterns, belief systems, attitudes, and mindsets that parasitize one's ability to think properly and accurately. Once these mind viruses take hold of one's neuronal circuitry, the afflicted victim loses the ability to use reason, logic and science to navigate the world. Instead, one sinks into an abyss of infinite lunacy best defined by a dogged and proud departure from reality, common sense, and truth.

—Gad Saad (2020, p. 17)

Abstract This chapter extends concerns made in the previous chapter and examines how constant exposure to digital media affects children's developing brains. In Australia, where over 97% of households with children have internet access, young minds encounter unprecedented levels of violence, addictive content, cyberbullying and radical influences. Research demonstrates that exposure to violent media can desensitise children, reduce empathy, and alter brain activity, particularly in prefrontal regions responsible for impulse control. The chapter provides insights into how screen addiction shares neurological similarities with substance addictions and correlates with increased anxiety and poorer psychological wellbeing. Relatedly, cyberbullying represents a modern evolution of

M. C. Nagel, R. Sharman, *Virtual Autism and Other Screen Disorders*, Palgrave Studies in Cyberpsychology, https://doi.org/10.1007/978-3-032-00803-9_7

traditional bullying, following children everywhere without reprieve, with particular impact on adolescent girls through relational aggression and social exclusion. Most concerning is how radical online influencers exploit vulnerable adolescents' natural identity-seeking behaviours through systematic deception, isolation and depletion tactics. The chapter emphasises how unrestricted access to digital content creates perfect conditions for exploitation of young minds ill-equipped to navigate these complex social environments.

Keywords Social Learning Theory • Violence • Desensitisation • Addiction • Cyberbullying • Radicalisation

Today's children live in a 24/7 media rich interconnected reality of virtual activity. In Australia over 97% of households with children under 15 years have access to the internet, with an average number of 7.8 devices per home; 99% of households with children under 15 years used a mobile or smartphone to access the internet, and social media is rapidly becoming the preferred news source among young people.[1] But what, precisely, are children being exposed to via these conduits? Could it be that many young minds are being 'parasitized' as described by Professor Gas Saad in the quote above and if so, might such pathogens of the mind be less than favourable for individual and collective humanity?

Of course there are many positives associated with engaging with the internet. Gone are the days when heated family arguments erupted over "What's the name of that actor?" or "What's the capital of Uzbekistan?" Screen devices bring with them a highway of information coupled with convenience of access. Unfortunately, such conveniences do not come without challenges and concerns. The dark side of this tsunami of data and ease of access has created a very different world for young people and by association is shaping their brains, minds and behaviour in ways we are only beginning to understand. And as explored throughout this book, we must continue to ask what are the potential effects of these exposures on a growing brain?

[1] Australian Bureau of Statistics, Household use of information technology 2018. https://www.abs.gov.au/statistics/industry/technology-and-innovation/household-use-information-technology/latest-release

Violence and the Developing Brain

For many years people have wondered about the influence of various forms of violent media on child development. When the television first entered people's homes in the late 1940s very few could afford them but by the early 1950s those numbers began to grow exponentially. When Neil Armstrong stepped onto the moon in 1969, millions sat glued to the TV screen to see this achievement. It wasn't too much longer that television began to broadcast for the sake of entertainment and titillation rather than news and education. As television became a medium for more that news, developmental psychologists began to scrutinise what impact TV was having on children, particularly if they were witnessing any forms of violence. Even the animated actions of Bugs Bunny and other popular cartoon characters became cause for concern. After all, what was stopping a child from copying Wile E. Coyote's incessant desire to harm the Roadrunner and drop an anvil on an unsuspecting sibling? In fact the concerns associated with viewing violence on TV screens has been justified with clear evidence that television violence can foster aggressive behaviour and cultivate a values system favouring violence to resolve conflicts.[2] It would seem that what we visually consume can impact on our behaviour. So much so that today, and within the parameters of Social Learning Theory,[3] the mantra of 'children see, children do' is used to push certain agendas and keep parents hypervigilant about their own behaviour in front of their kids. With recent advances in technology since the turn of the century, concerns over what is consumed via television screens has been exacerbated by the reality that children can now watch most things, anytime, in the palm of their hand. For example, while the use of screens, and in particular social media, to stream extreme violence is a relatively new issue, researchers have struggled to keep up with potential impacts of streamed acts of actual violence in real-time on the developing brain.

[2] Murray (2012).

[3] Social Learning Theory is the product of the work done by Professor Albert Bandura at Stanford University in the 1960s and early 1970s. For a fuller description of his work see Bandura (1962, 1977); Bandura and Walters (1963).

There are some things we are just starting to understand. For example, we now know that exposure to violence can lead to desensitisation, which can contribute to later acts of violence in adolescence.[4] Peer norms are also important here in that teens will tend to mimic the mood or context in which it is shared (horror and disgust versus amusement and sarcasm).[5] Such behaviours are well documented in the research literature and anecdotally observed by us as researchers and parents. Michael has a particularly relevant example that occurred when he was picking up his son from high school one afternoon.

Upon arriving at the school, my son told me that there was going to be a fight between two teen boys, one who was a Year 12 student and the other who had finished high school the year before. I was surprised to learn that the event was broadcast via social media detailing time and place … a park not far from the school. As a parent, educator and concerned citizen I felt compelled to do something to curtail the violence and potential for injury. Upon arriving at the scene was I flabbergasted at the number of students circling the two combatants who had started their battle. Equally astonishing was that most of the students were making a recording of the event with their phones and appeared completely oblivious to the violence unfolding in spite of the blood flowing from one of the boy's head and nose. This 'techno-voyeurism' only concluded when some informed teachers arrived on the scene to put an end to the ordeal. Those teachers were met with jeers and booing from students for stopping the fight. There was little, if any, sense or recognition of the violent nature of the event as students scrambled to post their videos presumably in search of 'likes' or other forms of digital affirmation. Such events lead us to speculate that peers sharing violent content for a laugh or any form of acknowledgement appear to provide a perfect storm of desensitisation and tacit peer approval for acts of extreme violence.

Watching a fight between teen boys is one thing but the impact of streaming violent imagery on children is quite another and varies depending on age. Younger kids may struggle to understand that another person holds a different, yet valid perspective to their own (developing Theory of

---

[4] Mrug et al. (2015).

[5] Fikkers et al. (2016).

Mind). Children may assume the threat presented in violent media is immediate and likely to affect them. They may also struggle to put rare versus common events into perspective because of their limited abstract reasoning.[6] Teenagers are still at risk of personalising and catastrophising the risk towards them and their peers in general, but are less likely to react with fear and anxiety compared to their younger counterparts.

In all, we have good reason to believe that continued exposure to violent acts streamed via social media can lead to desensitisation, with knock-on effects of lowered empathy and heightened fear and anxiety. There is also evidence noting that high media violence exposure alters activity in the brain. Researchers have found that when exposed to violent media, the regions of the brain used to control and inhibit behaviour, think through consequences and plan for the future (the prefrontal lobes) are effectively limited or in layperson's terms, switched off while those areas responsible for fight or flight become hypervigilant and ready for action.[7] Taken in its entirety we can surmise that a fearful person with lowered empathy is at greater risk of committing future aggressive and/or violent acts themselves in times of perceived threat—worth bearing in mind before believing teens become immune to the constant bombardment of this imagery. Equally worthy of consideration is the extent to which screen addiction feeds a craving for media violence.

Screens and Addiction

Remember the section in the preceding chapter about intermittent reinforcement schedules and how smart devices are set up to employ every trick in the book to get people hooked? What we didn't cover was the results of increasing screen time and social media addiction on addictive behaviours. This shouldn't really be a surprise to anyone who has ever spent time with any kind of addict.

Being addicted to something can lead to a vast array of personal and social issues. And while most people have heard of, or know of, someone

---

[6] Browne and Hamilton-Giachristsis (2005).

[7] Mathews et al. (2005); Wang et al. (2009).

who may have dealt with more familiar addictions, such as alcohol and/or drugs, there are others that may not be as widely known. For example, addiction to various aspects of screen devices is an increasing area of concern for those who work in the fields of child and adolescent development and psychology. Indeed, internet addiction and in particular addiction to gaming is now listed in the American Psychiatric Association's *Diagnostic and Statistical Manual of Mental Disorders (DSM-5)*.[8] This expansive volume of work is the 'bible' for describing mental health disorders and used by mental health professionals across the globe. Unfortunately, the relative newness of screen devices has not provided us with as much data as we'd like but a growing number of studies suggest that screen-related addictions are certainly worthy of concern. For example, there is some evidence emerging from MRI and fMRI studies that addiction to video games and social media has a similar brain base as any other addiction.[9] Importantly addiction, in and of itself, is often a precursor to other mental health challenges. This is especially evident when we consider that more time on social media has been associated with higher anxiety and being diagnosed with an anxiety disorder[10] while internet addiction has also been linked with higher levels of rumination, low self-care, social problems and poor academic performance.[11]

The depth of concern related to children and adolescents, addiction and social media extends beyond Australia's borders and is evident in extensive data samplings of American teens. Studies looking at changes across generations have found that the psychological wellbeing of American adolescents has dramatically decreased over the last 40 years, and this appears to be linked to an incessant desire to spend time on electronic communication and screens, including social media, while spending less time participating in non-screen activities (sport, homework, in-person interaction).[12]

[8] American Psychiatric Association (2013).

[9] Brockmyer (2014).

[10] Vannucci et al. (2017).

[11] McNicol and Thorsteinsson (2017).

[12] Twenge et al. (2018).

In short, the social media space is giving adolescents a warped perception of the world and the people in it. Digital representations of a false world are curated in a manner to have young people constantly seek out online utopias that they can copy. Fear of missing out (FOMO) and feeling inadequate against a backdrop of perfect lives/bodies is creating a sense of frustration that one simply can't 'measure up'. The fakeness of these TikTok/Instagram avatars is still lost on many teens, as they are more likely to believe at face value the imagery that's being served to them and strive to emulate what they see. As one of our older psychology students once quipped, "I'm not only jealous of other people's Facebook pages; I'm jealous of my own! Because in reality, that's not my life ...".

Cyberbullying

Most would agree that very few kids will get through life without encountering some form of bullying. We all remember the schoolyard taunts, the stealing/destruction of property, even the occasional pulling of hair, hitting and punching. However, yesterday's taunts or punch in the nose have been replaced with arguably more nefarious and psychologically damaging attacks. The major difference between then and now, that has been pointed out ad nauseum by many social scientists, is that once upon a time, the bullying ended at the school gate.

While bullying is a serious problem that has the potential for a vast array of physical and psychological harms, for many generations, bullying behaviour occurred in isolation settings and/or circumstances. Children could at least retreat to home, work, the local playground and physically distance themselves from the bully. This ability to escape provided victims with at least some space to process the events of the day or perhaps even an opportunity to talk to someone, strategise and come up with some solutions to the bullying.

But what now? Today's bully can follow a person home, in the car, to work, even into their bedroom at night, ever-present via a smartphone. Bullying is now happening in cyberspace, becoming more insidious, often with no reprieve for the victim. Cyberbullying is online harassment and can take many forms including aggressive behaviour, denigration, stealing information, insults, exclusion, impersonation, outing other's sexual preferences, breaking into accounts, hacking and creating damaging profiles or websites to defame another person.[13] Relatedly, research into sex differences in bullying provides further insights into how the traditional schoolyard thug is being replaced by the nasty little internet troll.

In one experiment, preschool boys and girls were given one valued toy to share between them while researchers observed their behaviours.[14] Boys who wanted to possess the toy tended to be very direct in their attempts to obtain the toy, either asking for it or snatching it. And I think we all know that, if not mediated by an adult, snatching can very quickly turn into a slap, hit or punch. Girls, on the other hand, tended to be more passive-aggressive and instead bullied by exclusion i.e., ignoring the girl with the wanted toy and playing their own game. Eventually the girl with the toy gave it up in order to be included in the group.

Fast forward to the teenage years and these favoured styles of bullying persist. By adolescence, the researchers noted that in an online context, bullying by exclusion or the spreading of malicious rumours (perhaps with doctored photos and the like) is on the rise and remains more prevalent for female targets. In other words, the modern bully is adapting their tactics to the new digital playground.

Bullying by exclusion also appears to more dramatically impact females, with teenage girls far more vulnerable to its effects. For psychologists this is not entirely surprising given the plethora of evidence noting that aggression in females is typically relational in nature and utilises exclusion, ignoring or the silent treatment, name calling, taunting, alliance building, shaming, gossip/rumour spreading and the desire to inflict reputational damage.[15] The psychological stress associated with this type of bullying can often lead to an array of other problems including eating and identity disorders, self-harm and mutilation or in extreme circumstances suicide.

[13] Moreno and Kota (2014).

[14] Marengo et al. (2018).

[15] Nagel (2021).

Suicide in younger girls is becoming more prominent with mental health and medical practitioners pointing an accusatory finger at social media as the background culprit. At a recent conference we attended, a leading paediatrician commented that seeing a suicidal nine-year-old used to be a rare and shocking event, but nowadays she was no longer "even surprised". Indeed, in their submission to the Human Rights Commission regarding suicidal behaviour in children, CYMHS (Child and Youth Mental Health Service) noted that thwarted belongingness (unmet desire for connection with others) was one of the more dangerous precursors to suicidal ideation.[16]

In all, violence via the internet is both transparent (live streamed acts that have become a source of entertainment); as well as pernicious (passive aggressive bullying). The oft mentioned several degrees of separation of being an internet troll tucked safely behind a screen rather that saying something false, malicious and nasty direct to a person's face, is driving down empathy for victims/targets, and ratcheting up entertainment value for the troll. One on one this is bad enough, but what happens when people are targeted online by a group for a more strategic purpose?

Radical Influences

While some of the challenges noted earlier may not be terribly unfamiliar to most, there is now a newer phenomenon with links to cyberspace sweeping the media pages and evident when a teen is caught doing something catastrophically awful. This phenomenon, referred to as "radicalisation" first started to be bandied about in the context of Islamic youth plotting or indeed carrying out terrorist activities. Since then, it has been widened to incorporate a range of criminal activities where teens are plotting or doing actual harm to others and using screen devices as tools for such activities.

[16] Submission by CYMHS for the Human Right's Commission's examination of intentional self-harm and suicidal behaviour in children and young people, June 2014 https://humanrights.gov.au/sites/default/files/Submission%20131%20-%20Child%20and%20Youth%20Mental%20Health%20Service,%20Children's%20Health%20Queensland.pdf

Just before we completed the manuscript of this book Netflix dropped one of its highest-ranking series on its viewing customers. *Adolescence*, a fictional account of a young boy radicalised by "manosphere" philosophies leading to him stabbing a female classmate who rejected his sexual interest became fodder for much speculation, conversation and condemnation. The fact this series skyrocketed immediately to success demonstrated how well all too many people resonated with the anxieties of parenting and adolescence. Emerging from this four-part series was much discussion around why some teens are particularly vulnerable to outside influences and in rare cases even inspired to commit acts of violence against others as a result? There are a number of plausible hypotheses to answer this question, but we'll focus on some well-established psychological mechanisms that may be at play here and pertinent to this chapter. From an evolutionary perspective, separating from parents, developing an autonomous identity and finding a "tribe" is imperative for survival of the species. Somewhat brutally, by the time you are an adolescent your parents' "day" is on the way out, and you are the new generation on the way to independence. Being able to relate to same age peers who will one day be your colleagues, friends and hopefully romantic partners is necessary for you to forge your own generational culture, pair bond and (brutally) breed. This is the way the human species has survived for millennia.

Identity formation, as discussed in Chap. 6, has long been considered the "core" business of adolescence. Who are you? What are your strengths and weaknesses? Your values, your personality, what do you bring to the table to help this new generation you are helping to form? To reconcile these questions, teens go through a process of trying on a number of different "hats" as they progress through forming their own identity. This process can drive parents quite mad—ironically these are the same parents who have conveniently forgotten their own foibles during this stage!

For those who can reflect honestly and without rose coloured glasses, will recall having lived through their teens passionately taking up a "cause" or strongly aligning themselves with a particular group. Teens start to form cliques and crowds (or in extreme cases maybe even gangs) with like-minded individuals to learn and mirror their behaviour. It is of no real surprise to most parents that teenagers who are trying to develop their own sense of individuality suddenly become the most peer-conforming person on the planet! They follow fashion, ideology, group-based stereotypes almost to obsession. Many are familiar with the more common teen groups of sports jocks, nerds, mean girls etc., but some teens get more creative and go Indie, Emo, gender non-conforming—you get the picture.

There is nothing new in any of this, and as a part of developing a robust identity, teens need to "try out" a range of different groups/friends/ideas to find where they best fit. It is, however, this desperation to connect at all costs, and "prove" their active and valued membership of a group, that can put some teens in a vulnerable position. Moreover, there are plenty of grifters out there who understand this vulnerability only too well and seek to exploit it.

A simple example is of course marketers. The realisation that a surprising number of people are gullible enough to purchase a product (any product) because of brand name, or celebrity endorsement (rather than the quality of the product itself) must have surely come from adolescent experts. Imagine, for example, buying a car, because it has a logo on it or is associated with a film star; over and above whether the car will actually drive you from A to B reliably! This is surely a form of self-delusion? In the teen brain (which we accept a number of people don't seem to grow out of) displaying tokens or symbols of group membership (via a brand for example) is paramount in signalling that they are part of the "in" crowd.

Teens, with their developing senses of perspective, proportion and their desperation to fit in, chase whatever symbol of acceptance they can find (the "right" hairstyle, make-up, fashion etc.), that signals the group to which they belong. Now, it's one thing to roll your eyes at the latest fashions, or decry how much your adolescent wants to spend on make-up, but what happens when all of this becomes a whole lot more nefarious?

Adolescent males, in particular, are experiencing a sudden and massive surge of the male hormone "testosterone". This rather extraordinary metamorphosis not only facilitates a growth spurt with accompanying muscle, bone, organ development; but all of a sudden a boy's brain needs to manage a hormone that brings with it a stunning upshoot of sexual interest and aggression. Remember also, that frontal lobe (the region that makes clever decisions and can put the brakes on stupid ones) is nowhere near fully developed in adolescence. In fact it's a good ten years away from completion. So now you have an increasingly large human, fit and strong, with an immature brain and surges in a hormone that he has yet to learn how to fully control. This can make for rather a dangerous beast at times. Western society has most recently attempted to manage these potential loose cannons by putting them into sporting teams where they can act out their energy, aggression within a series of strictly enforced rules. This is actually incredibly good training for most boys, as they learn (via immediate consequences) exactly what they can and can't get away with, and they also get to test and appreciate their suddenly increasing physical strength.

But what happens to those left on the sidelines? What of those boys that don't "fit in" to the standard teenage groupings that help shape their identity? Unfortunately, the online world can act as a refuge for adolescent males who are having trouble finding their tribe not too dissimilar to how girls look for like-minded peers to share their thoughts and feeling. And once again, this unregulated space is awash with a variety of grifters only too eager to exploit the vulnerable, undeveloped adolescent male brain.

Now, enter the radical influencers. They usually begin by preying on the known insecurities of the vast majority of adolescent boys as their bodies rapidly transform into those of men. It starts with some gym tips, personal training, maybe just a snifter of pre-workout formula! Similar to the status brands flogging rubbish to insecure teenage girls, these characters very effectively hone their message to boys. If they also happen to belong to the boy's ethnic, religious and cultural background they have themselves an almost immediate captive audience. Any adolescent who, for any reason, isn't "fitting in" with actual friends, peers or classmates or other groups is at heightened risk of being captured by these con-artists. And shortly after offering some genuinely helpful tips or workout videos and the like and capturing the attention of adolescent male minds, the messages begin to turn. The messages now feed teenage angst of not being part of their current crowd (their school, clubs, family, society); and entice them to join their welcoming groups online. Be it religious extremists, manosphere operators—the tactics are the same—they mirror classic cult practices: Deceive. Isolate. Deplete.

Here is how your textbook cult, or in modern society online grifter/influencer, operates:

1. Deceive. No cult is upfront about what crazy stuff they're going to get you to sign up to. If any group blatantly advertised "click here to blow

up bridges" they'd get very few takers. As outlined previously they hook you in with a typically sensible and relatable agenda e.g., work-out tips. Then slowly but surely the truth is drip fed with increasingly questionable agendas. A slightly crazy (but believable) idea is introduced first, if you are persuaded to take it up, a moderately crazy idea is introduced next and so on and so forth. Remember Behaviour Activation Theory from an earlier chapter? If I can make you behave, I can make you believe.

Eventually you are so far in you fall victim to the psychological trap colloquially known as the "sunk cost fallacy". You've now invested so much into these crazy ideas, at the cost of time, money and maybe even friendships (see Isolate below), pulling back from them makes you look, well, crazy! If only you continue a bit further and a bit further you might finally hit the knowledge jackpot (and yes for those of you wondering, gambling invokes exactly these same processes).

2. Isolate. Your school friends, teachers and even family don't understand you. They don't understand the pressures you are under not fitting in. You need to separate yourself from them. Don't tell them anything, they will try to pull you away from your genuine "tribe", i.e., the online one you've just found. In fact, post online to your newfound group any and all attempts from school/friends/family to pull you back to reality and they'll helpfully give you advice on how to push them away even further. Your new tribe is your real people, those outside the online echo chamber are not.
3. Deplete. This is often an overlooked but tremendously important aspect of cult tactics. In some way, shape, or form (usually multiple) the group will attempt to "deplete" your resources. This is to lower your capacity to think, reason and escape. Depletion tactics can take many forms with the most obvious being money. Give the cult all your money, so you have none for your own resources and importantly, any escape plan. It also helps fasten the sunk cost fallacy trap. But it could also come in the form of food or excessive exercise (you need to lose weight) or sleep (you need to stay up overnight on this chat room for 10 hours). These are also ways of ensuring you remain firmly attached to the cult for any form of nourishment (attention and validation), and diminish your cognitive capacity.

So let's put all of this together. We have a young adolescent male, with an immature and still developing brain and mind, often trying to cope with surges of a hormone he hasn't learned to control yet that naturally gives a sudden rise to sexual interest and aggression. For whatever reason he isn't fitting in to in-real-life cliques and crowds in his geographic region. He goes online to find his tribe … and boy what finds he can make. Violence and porn are ubiquitous, and as an adolescent can rapidly become desensitised, and possibly even addicted, to both. If he is psychologically vulnerable, he will be immediately targeted by the plethora of online grifters only too happy to have gullible minions for their own personal agenda. Adolescents become part of a tribe and radicalised in doing so,

Radicalisation is a new term for an old problem. Cults, vulnerable persons, addiction and exploitation have been part of the human experience since day dot. But it's the ease of access we have given to the con artists that counts here.

Imagine an analogous scenario involving a similar age-old issue: alcohol. We've always had alcoholics in our midst, in fact if we go back far enough we even see certain percentages of primates who appear to be genetically predisposed to alcoholism![17] Realistically, however, we can't change the human genome. But imagine if we were to create a society where alcohol advertising was allowed at all ages, with little to no restrictions on actual access to alcohol starting from primary school age. Even worse, by adolescence your parents not only encourage access to alcohol (because it keeps you quiet and out of their hair) but even allow you to set up an entire bar in your bedroom! Now re-apply that scenario back to what we've actually done in the modern Western world with screens and social media. Open access to those things a young mind is not yet equipped to deal with or navigate.

Summary

Chapter 7 extended concerns made in the previous chapter and examined how constant exposure to digital media affects children's developing brains. In Australia, where over 97% of households with children have

[17] Higley (1995).

internet access, young minds encounter unprecedented levels of violence, addictive content, cyberbullying and radical influences. Research demonstrates that exposure to violent media can desensitise children, reduce empathy, and alter brain activity, particularly in prefrontal regions responsible for impulse control. The chapter provided insights into how screen addiction shares neurological similarities with substance addictions and correlates with increased anxiety and poorer psychological well-being. Relatedly, cyberbullying represents a modern evolution of traditional bullying, following children everywhere without reprieve, with particular impact on adolescent girls through relational aggression and social exclusion. Most concerning is how radical online influencers exploit vulnerable adolescents' natural identity-seeking behaviours through systematic deception, isolation and depletion tactics. The chapter emphasised how unrestricted access to digital content creates perfect conditions for exploitation of young minds ill-equipped to navigate these complex social environments.

Bibliography and Further Reading

American Psychiatric Association (2013). *Diagnostic and Statistical Manual of Mental Disorders (DSM-5) – 5th Edition*. American Psychiatric Association Publishing.

Bandura, A. (1962). *Social Learning Through Imitation*. University of Nebraska Press.

Bandura, A. (1977). *Social Learning Theory*. Prentice Hall.

Bandura, A., & Walters, R.H. (1963). *Social Learning and Personality Development*. Holt, Rinehart & Winston Inc.

Brockmyer, J.F. (2014). Video games. In V.C. Strasburger, B.J. Wilson & A.B Jordan (Eds.), *Children, Adolescents and the Media – Third Edition*, (pp. 457–486). Sage.

Browne, K.D. & Hamilton-Giachristsis, C. (2005). The influence of violent media on children and adolescents: A public-health approach. *The Lancet*, 365(9460), 702–710. https://doi.org/10.1016/S0140-6736(05)17952-5

Fikkers, K.M., Piotrowski, J.T., Lugtig, P. & Valkenburg, P.M. (2016). The role of perceived peer norms in the relationship between media violence exposure and adolescents' aggression. *Media Psychology*, 19(1), 4–26. https://doi.org/10.1080/15213269.2015.1037960

Higley, J.D. (1995). Primates in alcohol research. *Alcohol Health Research World*, 19(3), 213–216. PMCID: PMC6875760 PMID:31798031

Marengo, D., Longobardi, C., Fabris, M.A., & Settanni, M. (2018). Highly-visual social media and internalizing symptoms in adolescence: The mediating role of body image concerns. *Computers in Human Behavior, 82*, 63–69. https://doi.org/10.1016/j.chb.2018.01.003.

Mathews, V.P., Kronenberger, W.G., Wany, Y., Lurito, J.T., Lowe, M.J. & Dunn, D.W. (2005). Media violence exposure and frontal lobe activation measured by functional magnetic resonance imaging in aggressive and non-aggressive adolescents. *Journal Of Computer Assisted Tomography*, 29(3), 287–292. https://doi.org/10.1097/01.rct0000162822.46958.33

McNicol, M.L., & Thorsteinsson, E.B. (2017). Internet addiction, psychological distress, and coping responses among adolescents and adults. *Cyberpsychology, Behavior and Social Networking, 20*(5), 296–304. https://doi.org/10.1089/cyber.2016.0669.

Moreno, M. & Kota, R. (2014). Social media. In V.C. Strasburger, B.J. Wilson & A.B Jordan (Eds.), *Children, Adolescents and the Media – Third Edition*, (pp. 435–456). Sage.

Mrug, S., Madan, A. & Windle, M. (2015). Emotional desensitization to violence contributes to adolescents' violent behaviour. *Journal of Abnormal Child Psychology*, 44, 75–86. https://doi.org/10.1007/s10802-015-9986-x

Murray, J.P. (2012). Children and media violence: Behavioural and neurological effects of viewing violence. In W. Warburton & D. Braunstein (Eds.), Growing Up Fast and Furious (pp. 34–55). The Federation Press.

Nagel, M.C. (2021). *It's A Girl Thing: Understanding the Neuroscience Behind Educating and Raising Girls*. Amba Press.

Saad, G. (2020). *The Parasitic Mind: How Infectious Ideas Are Killing Common Sense*. Regnery Publishing.

Twenge, J.M., Joiner, T.E., Rogers, M.L., & Martin, G.N. (2018). Increases in depressive symptoms, suicide-related outcomes, and suicide rates among U.S. adolescents after 2010 and links to increased new media screen time. *Clinical Psychological Science, 6*(1), 3–17. https://doi.org/10.1177/2167702617723376.

Vannucci, A., Flannery, K.M., & Ohannessian, C.M. (2017). Social media use and anxiety in emerging adults. *Journal of Affective Disorders, 207*, 163–166. https://doi.org/10.1016/j.jad.2016.08.040

Wang, Y., Mathews, V.P., Kalnin, A.J., Mosier, K.M., Dunn, D.W., Saykin, A.J. & Kronenberger, W.G. (2009). Short term exposure to violent video game induces changes in frontolimbic circuitry in adolescents. *Brain Imaging and Behaviour*, 3, 38–50. https://doi.org/10.1007/s11682-008-9058-8

8

Misplaced Love, Lust and Intimacy

For the first time in history, children are growing up whose earliest sexual imprinting derives not from a living human being, or fantasies of their own … the sexuality of children has begun to be shaped in response to cues that are no longer human. Nothing comparable has ever happened in the history of our species … they are being imprinted with a sexuality that is mass-produced, deliberately dehumanizing and inhuman.
—*Naomi Wolf,* The Beauty Myth

Abstract This chapter explores the evolutionary roots of human bonding and how modern digital influences are reshaping intimate relationships. Beginning with evidence of an ancient human population bottleneck that may have catalysed the development of Theory of Mind—our unique ability to understand others' perspectives—the text examines how this cognitive adaptation forms the foundation of love and pair-bonding essential to human survival.

The discussion then pivots to contemporary challenges, particularly how widespread pornography exposure is distorting young people's understanding of sexuality and intimacy. Early exposure to unrealistic, often aggressive sexual content creates disconnects between fantasy and

M. C. Nagel, R. Sharman, *Virtual Autism and Other Screen Disorders*, Palgrave Studies in Cyberpsychology, https://doi.org/10.1007/978-3-032-00803-9_8

reality, especially problematic for developing adolescent brains. The chapter also highlights concerning trends: anatomical desensitisation, consent confusion, and communication breakdowns between males and females with different evolutionary priorities and social skill levels.

The chapter concludes by examining the "incel" phenomenon and how social environments that shield individuals from necessary feedback can create adults unable to navigate real-world relationships, perpetuating cycles of social isolation and resentment in an increasingly digital world where authentic connection skills are more vital than ever.

Keywords Cybersex • Pornography • Theory of Mind • Assortative mating • Involuntary celibates (incels)

What's Love Got To Do With It?

What is love? How do we find the "one", and how do we progress relationships from interest, to friendship to romantic and sexual love? This quest has intrigued writers, philosophers, artists and everyday lay people since the dawn of time. To help us better understand the meanderings of thoughts around this topic let's go back quite some time—approximately 800,000 years ago in fact.

Evolutionary scientists have now analysed enough of our collective DNA to establish that nearly a million years ago humans were pushed to the brink of extinction. As few as 1000 humans may have been left on earth in what is referred to as a "population bottleneck".[1] This suggests that at some level we are most likely all related to each other! 1000 does not leave too many degrees of separation—so remember that the next time you're annoyed with your neighbour, go back far enough and you will find they're probably your distant cousin.

DNA relations aside, evolutionary psychologists have speculated that it may have been this catastrophe that compelled the development of what we have been discussing throughout this book: Theory of Mind.

[1] Hu et al. (2023).

Think about it, very small tribes of humans huddled against the outside forces of climate, predators, impoverished conditions and only a few of them to fight for survival would likely require an ability to sense how another might think, act and feel.

Some psychologists have pointed out that those humans who were able to better understand one another, work together, perhaps form survival bonds with other tribes and develop empathy for their fellow human (thereby increasing their chances of survival) may have been the very catalyst for this most extraordinary and unique cognitive characteristic known only to humans. Consider also that most humans form unbreakable bonds with one another, and most importantly their infant children who, compared to other mammals, are utterly helpless and dependent on full parental care. Was this the rudimentary, biological basis of what we now call "love"?

Love is not just a strong feeling or even motivational pattern, it may in fact, be absolutely crucial to our species survival. This is probably why, in spite of fast and quite radical social changes across the last 100 or so years, pair-bonding between couples remains the overwhelmingly dominant preferred relationship style across the globe.

So how do we create the bonds, that take us through friendship and affiliations, all the way to a concrete pair-bonding?

Social penetration theory (SPT) posits that the key to building intimacy is information transfer. Now that sounds rather bland, but when we unpack this, SPT talks about a series of self-revelations. Recall our discussion of the movie *Avatar* in Chap. 6 where we note how we exchange information and "reveal" our character bit by bit to those around us. The people who like what they see engage in this reciprocal revelation. And slowly but surely a bond is created. These people become our friends. Now throw in some lizard hormones and sexual chemistry, and one of those friends may even become our chosen "one". A romantic and sexual bond is formed, and children may even be born from it.

This is the way our species survived that catastrophe nearly one million years ago, and this is the way we will continue to prosper.

Cybersex

So, what then, are we to make of modern sexual practices? This almost needs no introduction but, to set the scene as it were, pornography is readily available on the internet with one source describing 12% of all websites as pornographic and 25% of all searches being for porn.[2] It also appears that at least one quarter of adolescents have unintentionally been exposed to online pornography and many of the unintended viewers are distressed by the exposure.[3] We would contend that unlike previous generations who might have had to hunt for some form of pornography such as a Playboy magazine, young people today can not only simply access pictures and videos online but also live channels for mutual titillation. In 1991, the year the 'World Wide Web went online, there were fewer than 90 different adult magazines published in the United States. Six years later there were roughly 900 pornography sites on the Web and in 2012 the software program CYBERsitter was blocking 2.5 million adult web sites.[4] One can only wonder what the numbers are now but regardless, access to such a cornucopia of online sexual content by children and teens is not advantageous for health socio-emotional development.

While there are a myriad of issues associated with pornography, one that is understood by most, is that sex in pornography is depicted as wholly disconnected from a caring relationship, instead presenting a variety of contexts with largely impossible poses; positions that are best for camera angles, and not for human anatomy! Such depictions essentially teach adolescents how to 'do it like they do on the Discovery channel' which then leads to unrealistic expectations and beliefs about sexual encounters and sexual intimacy.

By way of example, the excellent documentary film *Love and Sex in an Age of Pornography* included interviews with several teenagers about their sexual development in the context of digital porn exposure; many of

[2] Buchholz (2019).

[3] Mitchell et al. (2003).

[4] Ogas and Gaddam (2012).

whom described near-unbelievable sexual encounters that had been influenced by porn.[5] One male teen described losing his virginity:

> First time I had sex, cause I'd watched so much porn ... I thought all chicks dig this, all chicks want this done to them, all chicks want it up here, all chicks love it there. I tried all this stuff and yeah ... it went ... bad ...

For most adults this level of inability to separate fantasy from reality seems incredulous but remember that the adolescent brain does not function like that of an adult. A sophisticated 'Theory of Mind' is still developing and, as the opening quote of this chapter reminds us, what are adolescents learning from?

Let's go back to some brain basics. The average age of first exposure to pornography is 11 years, and at this age the mind of a child is genuinely unable to separate reality from fantasy. This is why younger kids often become scared in films and why an M rating is set at 15 years. Now we throw in some 'classical conditioning'. The young adolescent and their genitals become aroused by unrealistic, often violent and degrading images of sexual contact, separated from any kind of relational interaction. The bodies are all airbrushed and perfect. Labiaplasty, unheard of in previous generations, is one of the fastest-growing cosmetic procedures! Even nipple-resizing is now all the go. And we think most readers already know the average male penis is not nine inches erect—an apparently standard requirement for male porn actors. So the young adolescent brain becomes 'wired' for an attraction towards impossible bodies, with even more impossibly proportioned genitalia.

It is important to note here, that one of the most fundamental differences in terms of arousal is that males are more aroused by visual cues, and females by psychological cues. From an evolutionary perspective, visual cues convey information about health, fertility and youth while psychological cues provide information about a male's stability, commitment, social status, competence and kindness; males look to procreate, females look for material resources and stability to ensure the survival of their offspring. Perhaps this is why romance publishing often generates

[5] Corlett and Crabbe (2013).

more income than online porn. Not too hard to believe given that the 2011 bestseller *Fifty Shades of Grey* sold more than 150 million copies by the end of 2017 and had been translated into 52 different languages.[6] Prior to that Margaret Mitchell's only book, the wartime romance between Rhett and Scarlett in *Gone with the Wind* remained the world's bestseller for decades. And we have both lost count as to how many iterations Jane Austen's *Pride and Prejudice* has undergone in print, film and TV. It should not come as a surprise then, that females are not the largest consumers of online porn and males are increasingly accessing it at a younger and younger age.

Given males are visually aroused and the more voracious users of porn, young boys are particularly vulnerable to developing a slew of strange ideas as to what sex should look like. Giving rise (pun intended) to a new anatomical phenomenon, known as 'death grip'. The adolescent male masturbates to the imagery they see in pornography, essentially desensitising their penis over time. When they finally have the opportunity to encounter a real body, the mouth or vagina of that person doesn't even register as noticeable sensation for the male. About the only 'cure' for death grip is a total porn/masturbation ban, so the male brain and penis can recalibrate to an actual human being.[7]

Aside from being desensitised to the real world by watching a virtual one, 100% of 15-year-old males and 80% of 15-year-old females report that they have been exposed to violent, degrading online pornography, usually before they have had a sexual experience themselves. Nearly 90% of the scenes viewed included acts of physical aggression and nearly half-verbal aggression.[8] Relatedly, porn misrepresents pleasure, as the actors frequently pretend they are enjoying uncomfortable, painful or humiliating sexual acts. For example, it is well known that over 90% of females require clitoral stimulation to achieve sexual pleasure and/or orgasm, yet a recent British survey demonstrated nearly one-third of males could not accurately locate or label this rather vital part of sexual anatomy in

[6] See Johnson (2013); Schaub (2017).
[7] Jammel (2024).
[8] Horvath et al. (2013).

females![9] Go back to the example we gave at the beginning of this section of the teenage male who thought his first-time sexual partner would just love it if he roughly shoved everything into every orifice, and suddenly this makes sense. Online porn renders adolescent males with an inability to engage in authentic intimacy by providing them with continued virtual fallacies.

What of the girls in all of this? Another fascinating study examined certain pornographic trends that are inherently painful and unlikely to cause pleasure. Unless you've been off the grid and in the woods for the last ten years, you've probably seen or heard about the rise and rise of anal sex depictions in pornography. Interestingly, males have a prostate gland that can be stimulated internally via the anus, so there is an anatomical reason why some men might enjoy this sexual practice. However, females have no such gland and therefore the anatomical benefits to women engaging in anal sex are somewhat questionable.

Research by our own team recently investigated the rise of "unpleasant sex" from both females and their treating doctor's perspective. So prevalent was the mention of anal sex as problematic from the recipient as well as their treating physician's point of view, it merited its own theme in the study.[10] Furthermore, a British study concluded that young people have now normalised coercive and painful anal sex, with the young people themselves mainly reporting they wanted to copy what they saw in porn.[11]

We need to stress that we are not trying to 'kink-shame' anyone here. Adults are more than welcome to do whatever floats their boat! The issue, once again, is how do teenagers differentiate between fantasy and reality? How do young adults ensure they are communicating honestly and effectively their likes/dislikes and respectfully negotiate sexual boundaries? And what happens when those likes have been shaped and heavily reinforced by pornography rather than experience, with little regard for anatomical realties?

Expectations of females are rather challenging when it comes to intimacy in the twenty-first century. The pressure on young women to look

[9] El-Hamamsy et al. (2022).

[10] Sharman et al. (2024).

[11] Marston and Lewis (2014).

a certain way, possess 'perfect' genitals, and engage in sex acts that are inherently painful/uncomfortable with partners who have little clue as to the pleasure centres of their anatomy, is testing the mettle of this generation. Imagine being in a so-called loving relationship with someone who is clueless, clumsy or worse, keen to hurt you during sexual contact? It's no wonder teenagers and young adults are finding sex less and less interesting, with the current younger generation having less frequent sex than their baby boomer grandparents.

It is always important, when talking of issues related to children, adolescents and the virtual world to remember that the human brain does not mature until the mid to late 20s. This means that the immature mind is constantly being shaped and influenced by the stimulation the brain takes in every moment … *experiences matter*. As such, one final concern regarding the pornography-wired brain is that it fails to develop a sense of sexuality that is respectful, mutual and consenting. Because of this, we now find ourselves in a 'consent crisis', which is entirely predictable as social skills diminish or are hampered in the unrealistic virtual world of pornography.

How *Do* You *Know*?

Where do the circumstances and situations noted above leave relationship-building, and sexual relating? How do you 'know' a girl is flirting with you? How do you 'know' a boy really likes you but is too afraid of rejection to ask you out? How do you 'know' a person is initiating sexual contact, wants to continue with it, is enjoying it? Seriously reflect on these questions—how *do* you *know*?

The #metoo movement brought to prominence the difficulties that can arise when people get their wires crossed. Now we in no way wish to diminish the very clear and obvious acts of sexual violence and harassment that many women have faced, and continue to face in their workplaces, or indeed any places they inhabit. However, a number of these transgressions have left a few people scratching their heads. This is not an issue of "he said, she said", but increasingly we are moving on to "I thought/believed everything was going well". Again, how *do* you *know*?

Even long-time married couples can be surprised when they come to therapy that perhaps their partner's boat wasn't being floated in the way they assumed! Imagine again what can happen in short term, casual flings where one or both parties lack the experience and knowledge of the other person, coupled with poor intuition to pick up on discomfort or misinformed ideas around intimacy derived from cyber porn. The types of confusing scenarios noted above can be exacerbated by a lack of communication skills and the necessary relational sensibilities to assert true feelings about what is happening.

In our own research we not only asked women about their unpleasant sexual experiences, we also asked men.[12] Here was a quote from one of our participants that illustrates what can go awry in a heat of the moment series of assumptions:

> "Additionally, she tried to stimulate my rectal cavity, which immediately decreased my sex drive and made me feel awkward and confused. Although, I continued regardless out of courtesy".

Again, how *do* you *know* what you are doing is being well-received?

A lot of issues in this domain rest with a fundamental misunderstanding and an assumption that girls and boys have the same level of Theory of Mind. They don't. Many factors contribute to this but when girls assume that their discomfort or lack of interest should be obvious to a less mature male counterpart, this is not always the case. Couple this with the fact that we are seeing people lacking in confidence to negotiate boundaries around sexual interactions for fear of appearing inadequate or upsetting their partner and this often devolves into a lose-lose situation.

Young males on the other hand, have now started to react in a somewhat unpredicted fashion. Decades of research from an evolutionary point of view continues to demonstrate clear sex differences in the way romantic interest, or flirting, is both communicated and received. In general, women politely respond to male interest in a friendly fashion, which can be easily misconstrued by the male as her reciprocating his level of sexual interest. Evolutionary psychologists have been fascinated by this

[12] Weaver et al. (Under review).

"dance" between males and females and how it progresses towards intimacy, or comes crashing down in a heap.

Assortative mating is a term used to describe the well-known tendency for birds of a feather to flock together. To be perfectly frank, where you sit in the dating hierarchy tends to attract people at your level or below. In Australia we even have a slang for people who date above their league: "punching". Meaning you are dating someone who is considered more attractive and valuable as a partner than what you bring to the table, and therefore "punching above your weight".

The difference between the sexes in terms of how they prioritise certain attributes also comes back to evolution as alluded to earlier. Men, whether they are consciously aware of this or not, assess a woman's attractiveness based on fertility and breeding opportunity. Therefore, women who are of good breeding weight (neither too far under nor over), have genetic markers of good health (shiny hair, good skin, facial symmetry) and are typically younger (i.e., fertile) are favoured. Women, on the other hand, when looking for long-term potential will favour a man who will stick around to help her raise any offspring, so they tend to prioritise kindness, resources (to feed the chicks) and loyalty. These rules continue to apply regardless of whether you are voraciously child-free or outside breeding age. Your lizard-monkey brain remains a powerful influence throughout the lifespan.

Along with these biologically based criteria, socially we also know people tend to favour similarities in selecting long-term partners. So similar values, personality, social skills, intelligence, sense of humour, education, earning potential and yes, attractiveness and fitness. In other words, like attracts like.

So to be absolutely brutal about this (as evolution typically is), if across all of your attributes you rate about a 5/10, so long as you only go after other 5s or below, you should go on lots of dates and have lots of fun. If on the other hand you believe yourself to be better than that and go after 8s, 9s and 10s you will be rejected over and over. The same rules apply to both genders.

Research into sexual and intimacy development in modern dating practices, has noted that many individuals, particularly younger adults and teens, admitting they use the social media dating app 'Tinder' to gauge where they sit in the dating pool. This actually indicates very good insight. The teenage girl/boy isn't really sure where they rank, so they throw out their best advertisement online (photos, job, interests etc.) and see what they attract back. This gives them a sense of how they are being received by their gender of choice and what "type" of person they are attracting given their own attributes. Some of these young people have even told us they then have better confidence approaching potential dates of interest in real life, as they feel they have a better grasp of who they have a chance with!

However, what if your self-assessment and insights are way off. What if you lack the social skills to appreciate the polite fob-offs you are continuously receiving? You are convinced you are a 9/10. Unfortunately, everyone else ranks you as a 3. Additionally, women, in particular, will place a high value on social skills. So, what happens to the socially unskilled, moderately insightless male who has garnished his relationship skills online?

A new group of men calling themselves "involuntary celibates" or incels have exploded onto the scene decrying their lack of success in forming sexual and intimate relationships with women. It should come as no surprise to anyone that this group has a massive over-representation of autistics.[13] Now here's a challenge for you, the reader—put yourself in some difficult shoes and just consider for a minute, the predicament of the incel.

Imagine a young lad, we'll call him Johnny, lacking social-emotional communication skills is told throughout his childhood and adolescence that he is special and amazing (thank you Western education systems where participation awards thrive and everyone gets a get out of jail free card). He is growing up in a culture where he is continuously protected from himself and where any negative feedback is avoided or whitewashed less his self-esteem be damaged. Any socially inappropriate behaviour is excused away (maybe even with a diagnostic label). Johnny is not expected to change his ways or learn from his mistakes. In fact, he never really gets the message he is making social faux pas, instead the other kids are told he is special, and his increasingly weird behaviours must be tolerated and

[13] Broyd et al. (2023).

no one must ever react negatively towards him. Parents and so-called experts leap on this bandwagon decrying society's demands he should learn some manners, interpersonal skills and to socially "mask" (like the rest of us are expected to).

Little Johnny then heads into adolescence, noting that he has few friends at school, but lots of gaming buddies and social media avatars. Instead of bluntly telling Johnny what it is he says or does that rubs people the wrong way, he is increasingly treated with indifferent politeness by people who can't wait to get away from him. The invitations to hang out slow to a trickle to finally to none at all. Pretend excuses are made for his exclusion from events as a cover. He never realises this is happening, and is never given the option to learn why, let alone to learn how to do better. Because of his Theory of Mind deficits, he cannot work this out for himself. He needs help. Instead of feedback and practical support to develop better interpersonal skills, he gets a road paved with good intentions and a plethora of pathetic excuses to passive social exclusion, instead of uncomfortable but necessary conversations.

High school ends and shortly after his one or two school-enforced buddies send him a text message telling him they can't be his friend anymore. His 'friends' are relieved. He is devastated. His lack of real-life friendships and an over-reliance on social media throughout this most critical period of socio-emotional developmental means he has even poorer than ever emotion recognition abilities, conversational skills and social understanding in general.

Now he finds himself attracted to girls. Puberty and an influx of hormones will do that. On Instagram and Tinder the girls Johnny sees all seem so keen and encouraging. Scantily clad, sexually alluring and promising. Johnny repeatedly finds himself scrolling and liking much, but receiving little in return. At school he was told if he was respectful, and kind girls would like him and reciprocate. That never seemed to happen, but he figures he was shy and didn't know how to talk to them back then.

Eventually Johnny comes to the decision to make an approach to someone he is attracted to. Maybe to the girl at his work or his local barista who always smiles sweetly as she hands him his coffee. Instead of being nicely received he is heavily rebuked or worse, the manager is called to tell him to stop bothering staff. He is totally confused. He did everything he was told to.

Where does he find some advice on how to interpret these confusing interactions? Where he is most accepted and included. Unfortunately his acceptance, more often than not, occurs in a virtual world of gaming and social media sites. There he finds a whole population of young men just like him! They totally understand his predicament. In the real world he believes was just being nice and nasty females spurned him without giving him a chance. Why?

Having less than stellar social skills and by this age having no clue as to what he has no clue about, he fixates on concrete attributes. If he wants one of the hot girls, he needs to become taller, stronger, acquire more wealth and then the girls will flock to him. If you are sensing Andrew Tate vibes you are correct. And Tate is popular online with these like-minded males for good reason. The incels love him and embrace his lack of insight and shallow philosophy. All the while the in real-life interactions Tate has with actual females end in rape charges.

But just for a few minutes put yourself in their shoes. Look at what social media has been selling them for their entire developmental sexual period. Worse, society has clustered around them making excuses for their missteps and even waived away an unfavourable or anti-social behaviours entirely if they have themselves a diagnostic label.

This begins in early childhood where the "special" kid gets away with biting, and at primary school where he later gets away with meltdowns, absconding and assaulting teachers. Finally in high school, he is groping girls, sexually harassing female teachers and starting fights with the boys and once again his behaviours are excused by his "diagnosis". Not once does he receive a negative consequence and incredibly, in some cases, his victims are told they are the ones who need to develop more empathy.

Once Johnny leaves the cloisters of schooling his protections are chucked out the window. Having never had it explicitly explained what is wrong with his behaviour, paired without any consequences that might motivate measures of self-reflection and behavioural change, he rushes headlong into attempts at interpersonal relationships outside his former bubbles of protection and rapidly hits a brick wall of reality—people are neither willing nor required to put up with his crap. Once again reality fails to mirror the fake ideals he's fallen for online, and the well-intentioned reassurances from family and teachers, and he becomes disengaged, despondent or desperate.

Aspects of his early life where society has facilitated, enabled and excused Johnny's off-putting behaviours for years leave him in a quandary where he views the world as so tremendously unfair. He's never had the feedback he needed to understand why his behaviour is unacceptable. Even if he can't understand that feedback (because of his ToM deficits), he's never had the behavioural consequences to teach him quite simply "you can't do that, you need to change". Either approach would have been constructive, but at present all these young boys are getting is a wishy washy tut-tut with zero consequences, which is taken as validation for their increasingly dangerous beliefs.

Let us end this section with an actual example of a young adult one of us worked with. Late diagnosed autism (at the beginning of high school) primarily because he had no accompanying intellectual deficit. IQ testing revealed a level of cognitive ability fully two standard deviations above the mean, or in more local parlance, he was in the gifted category. Contrary to popular depictions of ASD (Rain Man, Big Bang Sheldon) this is actually the exception for ASD, not the rule.

This teenage Johnny found himself in trouble a few times at school, trolling people online and thinking he was "funny'. A few episodes of violent outbursts towards others were followed by deep and anxiety-producing remorse. The school did their best within their own confines. In the Australian system you are not permitted to "punish" a behaviour that arises from a diagnostic label. So no consequences, in turn resulted in no learning from his mistakes.

As he got older he learned nothing of social expectations because he was never permitted to receive feedback other than confusing conversations he didn't understand. The predictable dropping off of friends began. People not only rejected his invitations to hang out, but they also began to reject invitations from others to hang out if Johnny was going to be there. A few of his previous school enforced buddies made the point that if he was there, they would end up being "stuck" with him (as he couldn't socialise more widely) and likely expected to manage any outbursts or inappropriate behaviour (because that was their job at school). They just wanted to hang out with their mates in peace. They didn't want the added caregiving role anymore. So teenage Johnny became socially isolated with zero understanding of the reasons for his silent exclusion.

His one last friend standing (a long-term family friend) invited him to her 18th birthday party. This party would include family and close friends in an upscale restaurant. A couple of mutual friends expressed surprise and went as far as warning the birthday girl against inviting Johnny, but nonetheless, and in spite of their concerns, they accepted her invitation as well.

Everything was going fine, until teenage Johnny received the incorrect drink than the one he ordered. He! Lost! It! He began to verbally abuse the waitress, while fixating on the error, becoming increasingly agitated, angry and belligerent along the way. Several close family friends did their best to calm him while the waitress retrieved the correct drink and was promptly verbally abused again. The whole table, and restaurant, was left stunned.

The birthday girl and parents apologised to the waitress at the end of dinner (citing Johnny's longstanding and usual excuse of a diagnostic label). The waitress accepted their apology simply stating no one had ever spoken to her like that in her life. In the meantime, Johnny was completely undeterred and felt justified in leaving one-star reviews of the restaurant online and thinking the whole debacle was now hilarious.

The friends of the girl simply reacted with "we told you so". The wash up? Johnny was never invited to anything with his old friend group again. And he truly doesn't understand why.

This real case highlights the trajectory of children, adolescents and their parents who hide behind, or worse, weaponise a diagnostic label to prevent individuals from ever having to learn from their mistakes and improve their behaviour.

What is alarming is that this "approach" appears to be seeping into every aspect of society. Children are allowed to get away with increasingly appalling breaches of basic societal expectations, now, simply on the basis that they are children. Again, consequences are a bad word.

An example of how this perfect storm is now coming together at a population level is evident from the teaching coalface. Children in increasingly earlier stages of schooling are engaging in harassing, sexual and abusive behaviours towards female teachers in particular. This alarming behaviour appears to peak among young males in the mid-teens.[14] From a brain developmental perspective this makes a bit of sense. As they get older, and cleverer, the boys are still in the process of developing better empathy and communication skills. In a perfect, and dare we say normal,

[14] Schulz and McDonald (2024).

world the younger brain will still be struggling with these abilities, which is to be expected. It takes time to develop an empathetic, and by association moral, compass. In a world where social media reigns such development can be curtailed or even replaced with less than desirable outcomes.

So why this sudden rush of anti-social sexually inappropriate behaviour? Early exposure to porn, coupled with poorer and poorer social skills (emotion recognition, Theory of Mind, empathy, perspective-taking) and enabling parents eager to excuse their perfect child's outrageous behaviour are likely contributors to a perfect storm of misbehaviour. And once again, we often see zero consequences from the female teacher's workplace.

At the end of this chapter, ask yourself how intimacy-building and respectful mutual relationships are likely to be hampered by even minor impairments in fundamental socio-emotional human skills of relating to each another. The interpersonal skills relied upon for successful sexual "chemistry" are incredibly individual, private and nuanced. Taken together, online pornography and social media are an anathema to developing sophisticated and intimate relationships. Multiply that by 100 in the case of little Johnny who was born with ToM deficits in the first place. Instead of helping him do better, social media is validating and exacerbating his issues, whilst society at large turns a passive blind eye. This is creating a tsunami of boys with poor social skills, burgeoning sexual interest thanks to inappropriate porn exposure, and zero consequences for downstream bad behaviour. This is further exacerbated by a growing inability to listen, compromise and find consensus or a way forward; the topic of the next chapter. The only surprise in all of this, is that the situation isn't even worse.

Summary

This chapter explored the evolutionary roots of human bonding and how modern digital influences are reshaping intimate relationships. Beginning with evidence of an ancient human population bottleneck that may have catalysed the development of Theory of Mind—our unique ability to understand others' perspectives—the text examines how this cognitive adaptation forms the foundation of love and pair-bonding essential to human survival.

The discussion then pivots to contemporary challenges, particularly how widespread pornography exposure is distorting young people's understanding of sexuality and intimacy. Early exposure to unrealistic, often aggressive sexual content creates disconnects between fantasy and reality, especially problematic for developing adolescent brains. The chapter also highlights concerning trends: anatomical desensitisation, consent confusion, and communication breakdowns between males and females with different evolutionary priorities and social skill levels.

The chapter concludes by examining the "incel" phenomenon and how social environments that shield individuals from necessary feedback can create adults unable to navigate real-world relationships, perpetuating cycles of social isolation and resentment in an increasingly digital world where authentic connection skills are more vital than ever.

Bibliography and Further Reading

Broyd, J., Boniface, L., Parsons, D., Murphy, D. & Hafferty, J.D. (2023). Incels, violence and mental disorder: A narrative review with recommendations for best practice in risk assessment and clinical intervention. *BJPsych Advances*, 29, 254–264. https://doi.org/10.1192/bja.2022.15

Buchholz, K. (2019). How much of the internet consists of porn? *Statista*, February 11th. https://www.statista.com/chart/16959/share-of-the-internet-that-is-porn/#:~:text=Only%204%20percent%20of%20websites,might%20bring%20about%20new%20insights. Accessed January 25th, 2025.

Corlett, D. & Crabbe, M. (2013). *Love and Sex in an Age of Pornography* (Streamed online). Retrieved from https://www.kanopy.com/en/usc/product/love-and-sex-age-pornography

El-Hamamsy, D., Parmar, C., Shoop-Worrall, S., & Reid, F.M. (2022). Public understanding of female genital anatomy and pelvic organ prolapse (POP); a questionnaire-based pilot study. *International Urogynecology Journal, 33*(2), 309–318. https://doi.org/10.1007/s00192-021-04727-9.

Horvath, M., Alys, L., Massey, K., Pina, A., Scally, M., & Adler, J.R. (2013). *Basically...porn is everywhere. A Rapid Evidence Assessment on the Effects that Access and Exposure to Pornography has on Children and Young People*. Office of the Children's Commissioner.

Hu, W., Hao, Z., Du, P., Di Vincenzo, F., Manzi, G., Cui, J., Fu, Y., Pan, Y. & Li, H. (2023).Genomic inference of a severe human bottleneck during the Early to Middle Pleistocene transition. *Science,* 381(6661), 979–984. https://doi.org/10.1126/science.abq7487

Jammel, M. (2024). Death grip syndrome – What is it and reverse technique. *Fortius Health Clinic for Happy Healthy Live*, 27th November. Available at https://www.fortiushealthclinic.com/blog/death-grip-syndrome-what-is-it-and-reverse-technique (Accessed 14th April, 2025).

Johnson, Z. (2013). Fifty shades of grey release date pushed back to February 13, 2015 – Just in time for Valentine's Day. *ENews*, 13th November. Available at https://www.eonline.com/news/480515/fifty-shades-of-grey-release-date-pushed-back-to-february-13-2015-just-in-time-for-valentine-s-day (Accessed 17th January, 2025).

Marston, C., & Lewis, R. (2014). Anal heterosex among young people and implications for health promotion: A qualitative study in the UK. *BMJ Open, 4*(8), e004996. https://doi.org/10.1136/bmjopen-2014-004996.

Mitchell, K.J., Finkelhor, D., & Wolak, J. (2003). The exposure of youth to unwanted sexual material on the internet: A national survey of risk, impact, and prevention. *Youth & Society, 34*(3), 330–358. https://doi.org/10.1177/0044118X02250123 (Original work published 2003).

Ogas, O. & Gaddam, S. (2012). *A Billion Wicked Thoughts: What the Internet Tells Us About Sexual Relationships.* Plume.

Schaub, M. (2017). E.L. James has a new 'Fifty Shades": Darker from Christian's point of view. *Los Angeles Times*, 10th October. Available at https://www.latimes.com/books/jacketcopy/la-et-jc-fifty-shades-darker-20171010-story.html (Accessed 17th January, 2025).

Schulz, S. & McDonald, S. (2024). 'Not my boy'. When teachers are harassed by students, some schools and parents fail to help. *The Conversation*, 21st August. Available at https://theconversation.com/not-my-boy-when-teachers-are-harassed-by-students-some-schools-and-parents-fail-to-help-237122 (Accessed 14th April, 2025).

Sharman, R., Allen, A., van Niekerk, K., Coles, A., Manocha, R. & Foran, T. (2024). "What is normal?": A qualitative exploration of health practitioners reports of treating patients presenting with unpleasant sexual experiences. *Archives of Sexual Behaviour*, 53(10), 4099–4116. https://doi.org/10.1007/s10508-024-02994-3

Weaver, M., Allen, A. & Sharman, R. (Under review). Facets of unpleasant sexual experiences for heterosexual men. *Journal of Sex Research.*

9

My Way or the Highway: The Lost Art of Debate, Compromise and Understanding One Another

A vital part of what is involved in functioning as a human being depends on developing the imaginative capacity to see the world through the eyes of others. If we try to shield a particular group from experiences that help to develop this capacity, we risk doing them a profound disservice.
—Stefan Collini (2010, p. 41)

Abstract This chapter continues the exploration of the unprecedented impact of digital technology on youth development, moving beyond traditional generational criticisms. It explores how the first generation developing in a hybrid reality of physical and online environments shows concerning patterns in social-emotional development. As noted in earlier chapters, research demonstrates links between increased screen time and autism-like symptoms in children, while adolescents show declining mental wellbeing, diminished emotional regulation and weakened perspective-taking abilities. The virtual environment's emphasis on instant gratification and algorithmic affirmation fosters narcissism, tribal thinking and reduced critical reflection. Unlike the delayed gratification skills that predict lifelong success, digital immersion promotes immediate validation and black-and-white thinking. This technological experiment

M. C. Nagel, R. Sharman, *Virtual Autism and Other Screen Disorders*, Palgrave Studies in Cyberpsychology, https://doi.org/10.1007/978-3-032-00803-9_9

risks creating a generation with impaired identity formation, stunted emotional intelligence, and difficulty navigating complex social realities—effectively validating the term "Virtual Autism". These concerning developmental trends require urgent intervention strategies to foster healthy social-emotional growth in an increasingly digital world.

Keywords Impulse control • Delayed gratification • Emotional regulation • Emotional intelligence • Narcissism

What's Wrong with Today's Youth?

Whenever anyone takes on the task of writing and commenting on 'today's' youth they do so under the backdrop of a long history of older generations lamenting the perils and shortcomings of the young people around them. Such sentiments are evident in the historical works of Shakespeare, Mark Twain and others. Even some of Western societies' greatest philosophers were willing to have a fair go at the youth of their time. Plato, for example, was not very flattering in asking:

> What is happening to our young people? They disrespect their elders, they disobey their parents. They ignore the laws. They riot in the streets inflamed with wild notions. Their morals are decaying.

Not to be outdone, Aristotle posited:

> They [young people] have exalted notions, because they have not yet been humbled by life or learnt its necessary limitations; moreover, their hopeful disposition makes them think themselves equal to great things...they would always rather do noble deeds than useful ones: their lives are regulated more by moral feeling than by reasoning; and whereas reasoning leads us to choose what is useful, moral goodness leads us to choose what is noble. They are fonder of their friends, intimates, and companions than older men are, because they like spending their days in the company of others, and have not yet come to value either their friends or anything else by their usefulness to themselves. All their mistakes are in the direction of doing things excessively and vehemently ... they love too much and hate too much, and the same thing with everything else. **They think they know**

everything, and are always quite sure about it; this, in fact, is why they overdo everything. (Emphasis added)

Both Plato and Aristotle make fair points. They often do! And while their historical standing is enough to warrant some consideration, it is also noteworthy that roughly 2500 years ago both would offer the sentiments of many future generations beyond their time … including our own. In our personal and professional lives we contend that we are increasingly encountering younger and younger people who really do think they know everything, are often quite sure about that and themselves and tend to overdo everything. It is our experience that those of us who have been on the planet longer than Facebook have noticed some weirdness going on with 'young people these days' that is certainly beyond the observations of generations past.

Let's start by acknowledging that the current generation (the Millennials and younger) are participating in an interesting experiment in that they are the first to have developed their growing brains in an increasingly hybrid world of reality and online environments. Couple this with points made earlier about the developing brain. Specifically, experiences matter and the human brain wires itself according to the environment in which it finds itself. It is this remarkable capacity that has allowed human beings to thrive in strikingly different environments and spread in plague proportions across the world. Also, important to remember that our brains 'prune' away unnecessary neurons from puberty until we are in our mid-twenties, leaving only those useful for survival and functioning within our own particular social and cultural milieu. Therefore, humans can learn to survive along the equator as well as in the cold and forbidding environment of the North Pole. No other species has achieved this feat. Humanity's amazing capacity to survive in very diverse environments is directly attributable to our remarkably adaptive big brains that are shaped to deal with the particular environmental conditions we find ourselves in. We adapt, survive and thrive!

The same notions of adaptability can be applied to our social skills. Adolescence is the time when that over-emotional and somewhat reckless brain kicks into full gear to develop peer relationships that will drive future romantic pairings and hopefully form the basis of a new generation of philosophers, thinkers and leaders. A key question, then, is what happens in the developing brains of young people when those social skills are forming online? The true answer is, we don't yet know. But we have some recent research that gives us cause for concern.

Let's start by reflecting on critical points made in Chap. 4 and specifically with a reminder of the work of Romanian psychologist Marius Zamfir. Remember it was Zamfir who, in 2018, first coined the term that we have used as the title of this book—"Virtual Autism". In his clinical work Zamfir found children displaying characteristic behaviours of ASD and after tracking his patients for five years, noted a remediation of previously diagnosed autism if those children were simply kicked off screens and their parents trained in reciprocal play.

Then, in 2019 a meta-analysis of available studies concluded that there were clear links between increased screen time and poorer social skill development, however the authors noted causal pathways at that point were unclear. Heffler and colleagues were quick to follow with research that demonstrated higher television and video exposure at the expense of less time in-real-life play placed one-year-olds at greater risk of displaying 'autism-like symptoms'.[1] As part of the research, they asked parents fairly basic questions about their infants' abilities such as: Does your child look you in the eye? Does your child ever pretend? Does your child imitate you? Does your child sometime stare at nothing and wander with no purpose? Does your child seem oversensitive to noise?, and so on. Even in the first year of life, over-exposure to screens and under-exposure to in-real-life interactions made infants resemble toddlers with autism. There are now a plethora of individual research studies demonstrating a link between screen usage and autistic-like behaviours.[2]

Probably the strongest of studies helping frame our argument here was also presented earlier in Chap. 4 but worthy of acknowledging in this chapter. A Japanese analysis of over 80,000 children, tracked longitudinally, demonstrated that increases in screen time exposure at age one either ***doubled*** or ***trebled*** the risk of autism diagnosis by age three; as

---

[1] Heffler et al. (2020).

[2] Slobodin et al. (2019); Kushima et al. (2022).

screen time went up, so did the subsequent diagnosis rate.[3] Interestingly those results only held for male children, once again highlighting the interaction between both nature and nurture. That is to say people with a predisposition to developing a particular disorder (in this case males-autism) are more vulnerable to external triggers that may let that genie out of the bottle.

Such findings beg the obvious question as to whether these autism-like symptoms are reversible? Zamfir clearly demonstrated that they were, and earlier studies supported his experiences and findings.[4] However, the knock-on effects of stunted socio-emotional communication are yet to be fully realised, and their reversibility remains largely unknown. It seems reasonable to speculate that friendship formation, building strong social bonds and essentially playing well with others will be negatively affected. In the end, many aspects of wellbeing are likely to be diminished as children struggle to form and maintain the types of social connections necessary to act as a buffer to psychosocial disorders. *The Lancet* confirmed what we've all seen anecdotally—that mental wellbeing in adolescents has "declined considerably during past decades" and noted evidence of detrimental impacts of screen time on mental wellbeing that started at just one hour per day.[5]

Yes, we also acknowledge that we have spoken at length throughout this book about mental wellbeing in both adolescents and children. We have also looked at various aspects of development and disorders but here we want to focus on other aspects of human development and being 'human' that require real-life interactions. We are concerned that such interactions may be diminished or hijacked by the activities and time on screens which in turn, can lead to a number of other challenges. The first of these falls under our ability to control our impulses and delay gratification.

[3] Dong et al. (2021).

[4] Uhls et al. (2014).

[5] Khan et al. (2021).

Kids Love Marshmallows!

One of the most important developmental milestones, arguably, is that of emotional regulation. You could say that emotional regulation is an umbrella term covering such things as self-regulation, impulse control, delayed gratification, emotional control and emotion management. Simply stated, emotional regulation encompasses our ability to control all aspects of our emotional brain. Remember the limbic system matures sooner than our frontal lobes so being able to put the brakes on certain impulses, emotions and motivations generally improves with age and once again, through experience. As we mature and our behaviours are monitored and tempered by older siblings, family members and parents/caregivers we learn that 'no' means 'no', running out into a street can be dangerous, an extra piece of chocolate cake while yummy may not be good for the waistline and experimenting with illicit drugs has consequences.

The development of emotional regulation is not simply biology or a product of our nature. Sure, temperament and personality play a role but so too do social interactions that accompany attachment and relationship-building.[6] This is yet another reminder of the interplay between nature and nurture and the importance of the environment in shaping much of who we are and how we act in the world around us. Relatedly we know that adults can positively impact the development of a child's and teen's capacities for emotional regulation. Prior to looking at how that might be and how screens might impede on such development, an example of the lifelong role that emotional regulation can play on an individual is worthy of some exploration starts with a discussion around a professor and some marshmallows.

In the 1960s, researchers at Stanford University studied delayed gratification and impulse control in preschoolers using a very simple and yet elegant experiment using marshmallows. Led by Professor Walter Mishel, and in a controlled laboratory environment, these researchers would simply present preschoolers with a marshmallow with a small proviso. They told the children that they would have to step out of the room for a few

[6] Crugnola et al. (2011).

minutes leaving the child alone with the sweet treat. The children were then told that if they waited until the researcher returned, they could have a second marshmallow. However, if the child could not wait they could ring a bell, the researcher would then come back immediately, but the child could only have the original marshmallow. So, the children could choose immediate satisfaction or wait for a further reward if patient. Once the instructions were given, the researcher left the room, went to watch the child from an adjacent room with one way glass and let the games begin.[7]

Initial findings from this study noted that there appeared to be three types of behaviours demonstrated by the children. Some children managed to wait the entire time and gain the second marshmallow as a reward with minimal effort. Other children wriggled uncomfortably in their chairs and had to exert a fair bit of energy to restrain themselves to ensure they got the prize. And the third type were those children who did not hesitate to devour the marshmallow once the researcher left the room with some even getting stuck into the soft sweet treat before the door closed behind the adult. This made for some interesting hypotheses around several factors, but perhaps more intriguing were observations of some of these participants as they moved through school and life.

Over the next 40 or so years as life rolled on, the preschoolers who demonstrated greater impulse control and delayed gratification presented far fewer behavioural problems in schools and did better scholastically including having higher scores on university entrance exams; when it came to 'school' they did better than those who could not stop themselves from eating the marshmallow. As they grow older, they presented lower levels of substance abuse including alcoholism, lower likelihood of obesity, better responses to stress and suffered fewer stress-related disorders and demonstrated better social skills as reported by parents and friends. On almost all measures, the children who could wait for the second marshmallow were doing better later in life.[8] Those who couldn't wait as preschoolers were not only worse off comparatively, but also appeared to have different 'brains', colloquially speaking.

---

[7] Mischel and Ebbesen (1970); Mischel et al. (1972).

[8] Mischel (2014).

In a follow-up study looking at brain activity associated with rewards, the marshmallow test participants showed different patterns of brain activity when engaging in self-control tasks as adults. Those who demonstrated greater delayed gratification as children showed greater activity in the prefrontal cortex, the region of the brain that controls many executive functions including decision-making, while the ventral striatum, a region that processes desires and rewards showed boosted activity in those who could not wait to have a second marshmallow.[9]

Now there are many things that one could explore and debate regarding the studies and findings arising from the marshmallow test. That does not negate the fact that on almost every measure throughout life those who could wait for that second marshmallow did better than those who couldn't. This suggests that delayed gratification and emotional regulation play an important role for success in school and life. After all, if you cannot regulate your emotions and impulses effectively, how might you navigate much of what you do over a lifespan of responsibilities, commitments and relationships?

Have Smartphones Made Young People Emotionally Dumber?

What does it mean to be emotionally intelligent? Author, journalist and psychologist Daniel Goleman offered an exposition into the importance of emotional intelligence in 1995. His book, *Emotional Intelligence: Why It Can Matter More than IQ*,[10] was released that year and quickly became a bestseller in many countries with more than five million copies in print worldwide and in 40 languages.[11] Goleman's work has been influential in many respects and at its core argues that non-cognitive skills are important considerations for leading a productive and successful life. Among those skills, he asserts that self-awareness, self-management, social awareness, and relationship management are key competencies that need to be

[9] Casey et al. (2011).

[10] Goleman (1995).

[11] Schawbel (2012).

nurtured. And while his work is often used in terms of building leaders and fostering business productivity, we would argue that *emotional intelligence*, or the ability to understand and manage your emotions and the emotions of others, is a vital life skill, encapsulating emotional regulation and requiring specific opportunities to develop and flourish.

Now if we return to emotional regulation as a subset of emotional intelligence, it is noteworthy that the degree to which emotional regulation is a product of nature or nurture is not always easy to set out. We know that, from a nature standpoint, temperament, feelings of attachment, empathy and perspective-taking have some underlying aspects of innateness and biological timelines; as we grow older, and barring any substantive trauma, and as our brains mature all of these capacities should flourish. We also know that each plays a role in how we regulate our emotions and learn to control our impulses. Importantly, and here is the kicker, our experiences with others, along with boundaries and environments that are secure and predictable also play a substantive role in that developmental equation. Unlike IQ, emotional intelligence is not anchored in biology alone. Therefore, it is important to consider what might be happening to those developmental skills and milestones of young people who are spending too much time on screens and not enough time with real people in real-world contexts.

Generations surely change across time, and it turns out that contemporary researchers who have been studying generational changes are noting some consistent patterns. For example, there appears to be a generational decline in perspective-taking ability coupled with a greater sense of entitlement and increase innarcissism.[12] These changes appear to have begun at the turn of the century and been exacerbated with the advent of screens and handheld technology. We noted in an earlier chapter how the values of those who have been born and grown up in a world of screens and virtual environments have shifted away from community and social affiliations, to money, fame and image. It is important to recognise that these shifts are not simply the folly of youth but are also the product of a perfect societal storm in many Western nations where social media has created illusions, and delusions, of grandeur. Starting from

[12] Twenge and Campbell (2013).

'selfies' and postings on Facebook and Instagram to proclamations of being an 'influencer', a focus on self and self-promotion has fed an explosion of narcissism. So much so that people find themselves waiting to be liked because of their online posting of a picture of what they had for breakfast that day. And while that might seem like a rather flippant comment, there is nothing flippant about the fact that narcissism and a focus on 'me' leads to declines in prosocial behaviour, diminishes social connections along with civil engagement with others.

When a young person becomes obsessed with themselves, perspective-taking and empathy are the casualties of such thinking and identity formation. A focus on self makes it difficult to work through relational challenges and complex problems in real life. A focus on self fosters a deep desire to be 'right' and with the click of a mouse feed one's biases. Simply by logging on to social media a young mind can be fed a pile of misrepresentations by an algorithm designed to momentarily bolster their feelings or righteousness, validation and social inclusion. And this is done without any dissenting opinions and supported by a league of like-minded individuals who have been captured by the same algorithmic virtual magnet.

A further important consideration is when might the youth of today have opportunities for self-reflection, learning and mind-change while living in a 24/7 matrix of anonymity and misinformation? What might be the products of any deficits in scrutinising one's own thinking or considering the perspectives of others? Often, the results of such activities emerge online with ambiguous identities spewing black and white opinions, fiercely defended with little to no shades of grey, nuanced opinions or any open-mindedness. Ideas are often limited to a number of characters on a tweet or seconds on TikTok, compounded by poor attention and concentration leaving little room for deep and meaningful reflection and/or critical thinking. Not to be outdone, even mainstream media rarely affords any time for the sharing and scrutiny of differing ideas and instead falls into tribalism—someone must be right and others wrong. Remember also that this occurs in a virtual world where signalling one's virtue and seeking affirmation and belonging is prolific; a world very different from previous generations. A world also where bad ideas or silly meanderings of thought exist in virtual perpetuity.

Consider, for example, any embarrassing ideologies or beliefs you harboured across your lifespan. Especially recall those beliefs you held during your teenage years when your brain was still developing. What might the outcome be if you were to post such thoughts or photos online for all the world to see? Many a celebrity, sportsperson or politician has become unstuck when an old tweet, social media post or drunken blackface at a party has popped up thanks to the eternal lifespan of servers. People have had their reputations damaged, lost livelihoods and careers for posting something stupid as a teenager or young adult. They are often left to apologise, often to no effect, and ostracised or 'cancelled'. All we can say is that there but for the grace of good luck would go all of us.

Those, however, who earnestly believe they are in a position to cast a first virtual stone on any issue almost certainly fit into Amos Oz's definition of a fanatic in Chap. 6. Remember, the fanatic has no private life, no relationship, no warmth and is one hundred percent public with a desire to consolidate their belief system and force others to change!

Consider then, for just a minute—what is such a person's first response when attacked? To defend? That would certainly be the norm. So if they hold an idea that doesn't stack up well to analysis, but now they've blasted it out publicly, what can they do? Do they dig their heels in and defend further, or do they back down and apologise profusely for fear of being yet another victim of the cry-bullies? Either way, did the mobbing genuinely cause the recipient of online vitriol to reflect, ponder and change their mind? Or did it cement their position further? Or did the experience make them more mindful of presenting a public self that is totally at odds with their private self through self-capitulation—otherwise known as being inauthentic or a fraud? This is the virtual world young people find themselves in. A world where being one's true self is hindered by a desire to be seen, heard and self-indulged. A world where algorithms create environments for proclaiming one's importance and attacking those who disagree or make mistakes. A world where the errors or beliefs of the past are too often held through today's prism of judgement by those who would feign moral superiority.

The thought and behaviour police, especially on social media, are becoming increasingly voracious. Some Dr Seuss books have been withdrawn from publication due to pictorial representations once seen as permissible. (Those who don't understand the magnitude of this from a historical perspective might like to look up book-burning.) Sportspeople are being forced against their will to make public displays in favour of political positions. Regardless of whether they agree with said position or not, is it ever OK to force people to do so when their job is to chase a ball around a field? And ordinary people will quickly get online to note that they have jumped on a particular bandwagon lest they be singled out for not doing so. In recent times this has included being part of contested issues such as vaccinations or pledging support to one country over another in a distant war. And in an environment where online platforms and social media are omnipresent, this creates a significant problem for today's young minds. For many young people, who have a diminished capacity for looking at things from various perspectives due to an immature brain and a less than optimum environment, the road to speaking and acting without thinking and reflection is not only problematic for the individual but also for the social and cultural milieu in which they exist.

We live in increasingly dangerous times for free speech as extremists leak into surprising avenues of thought and debate to shut it all down. Again, even if you disagree vehemently with what is being said, what is the outcome of banning thought and speech? We already know that in most instances, you simply drive dangerous ideas underground where they fester, and their proponents become increasingly incensed by the message they receive that somehow, they are 'lesser' for believing them. Robust debates, even of unpalatable ideas, are the only way to air how people think. Attempted suppression often does little but give unpalatable ideas fertiliser to propagate further.

Martin Luther King Jr once said that *darkness cannot drive out darkness; only light can do that.* In our estimation, screens and social media are part of a psychological darkness. We don't yet fully understand or know what life on social media does to the developing identity, but we only need look to current events to see a range of psychological processes playing out in ways that while not unforeseen, perhaps were underestimated.

We contend that social media may be creating a form of identity 'stunting', that is, teens bandwagon into groups and become increasingly tribal instead of having the opportunity to genuinely develop their own identity. Relatedly, deficiencies in, or the lack of, perspective-taking, empathy building and a total unwillingness to engage in an idea or position that isn't the popularity bolster de jour, is shaping a generation of 'sheeple' incapable of critical thought and self-reflection. Moreover, following the herd is not an advantageous path for the developing brains and minds of young people.

If you recall from previous chapters, we noted how identity development is a key component of the psychological business of adolescence. This is where we decide who we are, what we stand for and start to question what we want out of life. It's actually a thrilling time, albeit not so much for one's parents! But what happens if that individual development is thwarted or hijacked? Remember also we have discussed the process of Behavioural Activation (if you behave it you believe it)? We bring these two important concepts to your attention once again and ask you to contemplate the outcomes of teens who find themselves leaping onto ideologies fed to them via marketing algorithms. The nature of tweeting and snapchatting is all about instant recognition and self-gratification. There is little appetite for thoughtful mulling of ideas and the development of critical thinking, let alone mind-change. How might teens learn to back away from publicly proclaimed opinions that are provided as fodder for their own beliefs? In the end, identity politics, accompanied by an unwillingness to hear dissenting ideas stunts healthy emotional development and by association social cohesion. Instead of making mistakes, rethinking, reflecting and analysing to forge their own identity, teens addicted to social media are lost in a matrix of narcissism, numb to the real world around them and unable to connect. A generation, who for all intent and purposes, is showing the less glamourous aspects of autistic impairments. The question then, is what, if anything, can be done to diffuse this and promote healthy development? Our final chapter helps to provide some answers to this important question.

Summary

Chapter 9 continues the exploration of the unprecedented impact of digital technology on youth development, moving beyond traditional generational criticisms. It explores how the first generation developing in a hybrid reality of physical and online environments shows concerning patterns in social-emotional development. As noted earlier, research demonstrates links between increased screen time and autism-like symptoms in children, while adolescents show declining mental wellbeing, diminished emotional regulation and weakened perspective-taking abilities. The virtual environment's emphasis on instant gratification and algorithmic affirmation fosters narcissism, tribal thinking and reduced critical reflection. Unlike the delayed gratification skills that predict lifelong success, digital immersion promotes immediate validation and black-and-white thinking. This technological experiment risks creating a generation with impaired identity formation, stunted emotional intelligence, and difficulty navigating complex social realities—effectively validating the term "Virtual Autism". These concerning developmental trends require urgent intervention strategies to foster healthy social-emotional growth in an increasingly digital world.

Bibliography and Further Reading

Casey, B.J., Somerville, L.H., Gotlib, I.H., Ayduk, O., Franklin, N.T., Askren, M.K., Jonides, J., Berman, M.G., Wilson, N.L., Teslovich, T., Glover, G., Zayas, V., Mischel, W. & Shoda, Y. (2011). Behavioral and neural correlates of delay gratification 40 years later. *Proceedings of the National Academy of Sciences*, 108(36), 14998–15003. https://doi.org/10.1073/pnas.1108561108

Collini, S. (2010). *That's Offensive: Criticism, Identity, Respect.* Seagull Books.

Crugnola, C.R., Tambelli, R., Spinelli, M., Gazzoti, S., Caprin, C. & Albizzati, A. (2011). Attachment patterns and emotion regulation strategies in the second year. *Infant Behaviour & Development*, 34(1), 136–151. https://doi.org/10.1016/j.inbeh.2010.11.002

Dong, H.Y., Feng, J.Y, Wang, B., Shan, L. & Jia, F.Y. (2021) Screen Time and Autism: Current Situation and Risk Factors for Screen Time among

Pre-School Children with ASD. *Frontiers in* Psychiatry, 12:675902. https://doi.org/10.3389/fpsyt.2021.675902

Goleman, D. (1995). *Emotional Intelligence: Why It Can Matter More Than IQ*. Bantam Books.

Heffler K.F., Sienko D.M., Subedi K., McCann K.A., Bennett D. S. (2020) Association of early-life social and digital media experiences with development of autism spectrum disorder–like symptoms. *JAMA Pediatrics* 174(7):690–696. https://doi.org/10.1001/jamapediatrics.2020.0230

Khan, A., Lee, E. Y., Rosenbaum, S., Khan, S. R., & Tremblay, M. S. (2021). Dose-dependent and joint associations between screen time, physical activity, and mental wellbeing in adolescents: an international observational study. *The Lancet. Child & Adolescent Health*, *5*(10), 729–738. https://doi.org/10.1016/S2352-4642(21)00200-5

Kushima et al., (2022). Association between screen time exposure in children at 1 year of age and autism spectrum disorder at 3 years of age The Japan Environment and Children's Study. JAMA Pediatrics, 176(4), 384–391. https://doi.org/10.1001/jamapediatrics.2021.5578

Mischel, W. (2014). *The Marshmallow Test: Understanding Self-Control and How to Master It*. Bantam Press.

Mischel, W. & Ebbesen, E.B. (1970). Attention in the delay of gratification. *Journal of Personality and Social Psychology*, 16(2), 329–337. https://doi.org/10.1037/h0029815

Mischel, W., Ebbesen, E.B. & Raskoff Zeiss, A. (1972). Cognitive and attentional mechanisms in delay of gratification. *Journal of Personality and Social Psychology*, 21(2), 204–218. https://doi.org/10.1037/h0032198

Schawbel, D. (2012). Daniel Goleman on the importance of ecological intelligence. *Forbes*, 1st August. Available at https://www.forbes.com/sites/danschawbel/2012/08/01/daniel-goleman-on-the-importance-of-ecological-intelligence/ (Accessed 23rd April, 2025).

Slobodin, O., Heffler, K.F. & Davidovitch, M. (2019). Screen media and autism spectrum disorder: A systematic literature review. *Journal of Developmental & Behavioral Pediatrics* 40(4), 303–311. https://doi.org/10.1097/DBP.0000000000000654

Twenge, J.M. & Campbell, W.K. (2013). *The Narcissism Epidemic: Living in the Age of Entitlement*. Atria Paperback.

Uhls, Y.T., Michikyan, M., Morris, J., Garcia, D., Small, G. W., Zgourou, E., & Greenfield, P. M. (2014). Five days at outdoor education camp without screens improves preteen skills with nonverbal emotion cues. *Computers and Human Behavior, 39*, 387–392.

10

Natural Buffers to Screen Disorders

…the digital age has stripped away certain critical and sanity-sustaining dynamics that once were prevalent and now no longer exist: We need experiences that nurture our ability to be patient. Instead, we have Twitter. We need real hand-eye experiences. Instead, we have gaming. We need face-to-face interpersonal social experiences. Instead, we have social media. We need nature-immersive experiences. Instead, we have some pics of nature on Instagram. That just does not cut it if we want to be truly healthy, strong, and happy.

—Dr Nicholas Kardarsas (2022, p. 229)

Abstract This chapter consolidates the preceding chapters, drawing attention to how excessive screen time displaces critical developmental experiences for children and adolescents. Human beings are fundamentally social creatures whose brains and wellbeing depend on meaningful face-to-face interactions. Play—particularly self-directed and dramatic play—is essential for cognitive, social-emotional and physical development. Yet screen time has dramatically reduced both social interaction and active play, creating increasingly sedentary lifestyles with documented negative health outcomes.

M. C. Nagel, R. Sharman, *Virtual Autism and Other Screen Disorders*, Palgrave Studies in Cyberpsychology, https://doi.org/10.1007/978-3-032-00803-9_10

The chapter highlights the therapeutic benefits of nature exposure, drawing on concepts like Attention Restoration Theory, Stress Recovery Theory, and biophilia to demonstrate how natural environments support mental health and cognitive functioning. Research shows that access to nature correlates with improved mental health outcomes, while time in challenging outdoor environments develops crucial competence and autonomy.

The authors argue that modern "safetyism" has contributed to children's increased screen dependence by limiting outdoor exploration. They recommend delaying device access until age 16, modelling healthy technology use, and creating boundaries that shift the balance towards real-world experiences, particularly in nature, to buffer against the negative impacts of excessive screen time on developing brains.

Keywords Play • Physical activity • Attention Restoration Theory • Stress Recovery Theory • Biophilia • 'Safetyism' • Nature

Livewired!

Setting up the basic building blocks of the brain and get it into the world! That was the opening sentence in the first chapter of this book. We thought it would be an appropriate opening for the last chapter as well. If you recall, Chap. 1 explored the basic building blocks of the brain and touched on how those 'blocks', in conjunction with experiences, shape our neural architecture and minds. Experiences matter and this book has focused on the potentially negative experiences on the developing brain associated with ever expansive screen device usage at home and in our schools. This chapter also focuses on experiences. However, the following pages are about those experiences that positively influence the developing brain and may buffer the screen disorders mentioned throughout the preceding chapters. An initial look at the importance of social interactions and 'play' introduces the type of experiences research tells us are critical. This is followed by the equally important context of experiences in nature. As you progress through this final chapter always keep the notion of a 'displacement hypothesis' in the back of your mind; if children and teens are on screens, what aren't they doing? We start this discussion by reiterating something we have noted in other chapters; human beings are fundamentally social creatures.

The importance of social interactions is evident from the first day of postnatal life to the day when one's life draws to an end; being with others is healthy and necessary.[1] Neuroscientists themselves have acknowledged the importance of thriving through our social identities. During the 1970s the concept of the brain as a 'social organ' emerged as researchers started to uncover that our biochemistry, anatomy, neuroplasticity and overall health are deeply influenced by, and interwoven with, our social relationships.[2] In terms of overall wellbeing, the impact of diminished social interactions has been well studied and linked to a range of negative outcomes.

It is widely known that brief forms of social disconnections can engage a range of negative emotions (such as anger and sadness), along with deficits in self-esteem and cognitive abilities. Prolonged social disconnection experiences, on the other hand, have been linked with an increased risk of depression, suicidal ideation and early mortality.[3] Consider, for example, solitary confinement for prison inmates has been characterised as torture by human rights agencies due to the likelihood of such practices creating severe mental anguish, contributing to existing mental illnesses or exacerbating psychopathologies.[4] For even the most hardened criminals, being isolated and alone can create a great deal of emotional distress.

You don't have to be in solitary confinement to experience bad feelings due to not being with others! Loneliness itself has been associated with increased odds of asthma, migraine, osteoarthritis, rheumatoid arthritis, hypertension, depression, anxiety and long-term mental illness.[5] Loneliness impacts negatively on the body and mind. And because this book focuses on children and adolescents it is worth noting the increasing recognition that the global pandemic, and its associated health

---

[1] Porges (2003).

[2] Carter (2007); Cozolino (2013).

[3] Pancani et al. (2021).

[4] Cloud et al. (2015); Reiter et al. (2020).

[5] Christiansen et al. (2021).

measures including lockdowns and school closures, demonstrated the detrimental impact of social isolation on young developing minds.[6] People who need people are not only the luckiest people in the world, but often the healthiest.

It should be evident from the points above that social interactions are important for all people. For children and adolescents this is not just important, but critical for all aspects of development and screens get in the way of this development. Young people thrive and show positive developmental outcomes when they engage with others. This is not to say that all kids will be happy with all other kids all the time, but the evidence is conclusive, social interactions are a necessary component of healthy development. We can see this in the earliest days of childhood as children learn to navigate the world through play.

Let's Play!

Eeny, meeny, miny, moe, catch a tiger by the toe. If he hollers, let him go, eeny, meeny, miny, moe. Sounds silly as an adult, doesn't it? One of the challenges when it comes to discussing play is that many are not fully aware of the seriousness of this endeavour. Some hear the word play and think this is something to do after the hard work is done, or that it is a reward, or that its place in schools is secondary to all things academic. However, for children, fulfilling the important need to engage with others as noted in the previous section happens when they play with their caregivers and peers. Peer interactions teach social competence, how to get along with others, whether someone is a friend or foe and one's place in ever-changing social hierarchies. Perhaps the greatest opportunity for peer interactions as a teaching tool for acquiring such information is 'play'.[7] Play is vitally important for young people and according to neuroscientist and primatologist, Professor Robert Sapolsky of Stanford University, "a child deprived of, or disinterested in, play rarely has a socially fulfilling life"

[6] Pietrabissa and Simpson (2020); Pavin Ivanec (2022).

[7] Sapolsky (2017).

and “the opposite of play is not work—it’s depression”.[8] To the layperson that might sound a bit hyperbolic but once you understand what play does, Sapolsky’s words tend to ring true.

Play and play behaviour have a long research history across many fields of study. It has been noted as an integral aspect of our evolution as it helps build the skills necessary for adaptation and survival. Most animals, and most certainly all mammals, engage in play behaviour and humans are the most complex and most playful of all species. The world-renowned neuroscientist and psychobiologist, Professor Jaak Panksepp demonstrated that play behaviours are part of the inner workings of the brain, indicating that play had an early evolutionary origin.[9] Our early ancestors played and because we still play today there must be something adaptive and beneficial for us in doing so.

For infants and children, play and playful behaviours are the foundations for early learning. Ask a child what they would like to do and most often their answer is ‘play’. Through play, all aspects of a child’s development are enriched. Creative expression, oral language, cognition, social skills, emotional regulation, and all manner of physical development are enhanced through play. Play is not simply an unimportant pastime. We know that different types of play, self-directed play and dramatic play for example, are particularly important.

Self-directed play is freely chosen. Allowing children to play on their own, without an imposed adult framework or interference, has been linked to better language and problem-solving abilities, better social skills, enhanced memory capacities and less stress in children. Dramatic play, however, is facilitated by adults who provide social scenarios and roles for children to adopt and guide them through activities and an understanding of the social norms of that role. A child who assumes the role of a police officer, for example, must behave in ways that meet that role and will often rely on private or internal speech to help define that role and govern their behaviour. They will have little conversations in their mind to ensure they look and sound like a police officer. They think about how they might act or what they might say while playing that role.

[8] Ibid., p. 205.

[9] See Panksepp (2004) and Panksepp and Biven (2012).

This type of play helps children to learn to curb their impulses. It also encourages self-regulatory behaviour and extends, among other things, oral language, phonemic awareness, letter recognition, familiarity with conventions of print and meaningful counting, numeral recognition and pattern recognition; some would refer to this as literacy and numeracy.[10]

There is so much more that can be said about the benefits of play for children. Quite simply however, when immersed in play children advance their physical, cognitive, communicative and social-emotional development. The benefits of play extend beyond the lab and scientific inquiry. Even the instruction sheet from Lego toys acknowledges that:

> When children play, they exercise their senses, their intellect, their emotions, their imagination—keenly and energetically … To play is to explore, to discover and to experiment. Playing helps children develop ideas and gain experience. It gives them a wealth of knowledge and information about the world in which they live—and about **themselves (emphasis added).** So, to play is to learn. Play is fun for children. But it's much more than that—it's good for them, and it's necessary … Play gives children the opportunity to develop and use the many talents they were born with.[11]

Stepping on Lego blocks can create excruciating pain for parents but may be a small price to pay for a child's development. Furthermore, we contend that *Eeny, meeny, miny, moe, catch a tiger by the toe. If he hollers, let him go, eeny, meeny, miny, moe* takes on new meaning when all the benefits of play are considered. Relatedly, when children play, they do so through social interaction that is pleasurable. The same can be said about play and adolescents.

Some might think that play stops when we reach a certain age. Perhaps it doesn't stop per se but rather it changes. As children move through adolescence they likely play less and do so in different ways given the demands of maturing into adult roles and expectations. However, although play may differ with age the benefits of play for adolescents mirror those of younger children. First, we know that play can support

---

[10] Lego instructions cited in Panksepp (2004).

[11] Nagel (2012). See also Pellegrini et al. (2007); Elkind (2007); Barnett et al. (2008); Diamond et al. (2007); Medina (2010).

learning in schools.[12] Second, and we think more importantly, play for adolescents provides further opportunities for social interaction and understanding how to navigate various group contexts. From an evolutionary perspective, play provides essential practice for future skills and relationships. And for some, play creates opportunities for flourishing and positive growth.[13] The same cannot be said for spending time on screens in the place of any form of play in real time with real people. We would argue that as we get older it is not the type of play that matters as much as taking the time to socially interact through play.

DON'T Sit Still!

Now while all this talk about play has offered some food for thought about the importance of playful activity, we'd like to quickly revisit part of the discussion presented in Chap. 6 before moving on; sedentary behaviour is not always healthy. We say always because reading and doing homework outside of school, are associated with higher academic achievement and positive feelings of self.[14] This suggests that there are qualitative differences in what young people do when they aren't doing anything active. However, at the core of this discussion is our belief that young people aren't moving enough, and screens are perhaps the most substantive contributor to that problem. Moreover, sitting still for long periods of time is not advisable and Japanese mythology offers an interesting analogy.

If you visit Japan, you are likely to encounter Daruma dolls or figurines. These dolls are generally round in shape and designed in a way that allows them to return to an upright position when tilted over. They are modelled after a fifth-century Chinese Buddhist monk, Bodhidharma, who became the patriarch of the school of Chan Buddhism in China. This form of Buddhism evolved into Zen Buddhism in Japan and because

[12] Johnston et al. (2023).

[13] Lockwood and Connor (2017); see also, Smith (1982); Bjorklund and Pellegrini (2002); Maslow (1970, 1999).

[14] Carson et al. (2016).

Bodhidharma is so revered for his perseverance and dedication to meditation the Japanese created Daruma in his honour.

One of the striking features of Daruma is the lack of limbs or any representation of limbs. These intriguing figurines do not have any arms or legs, and this is purposeful. Legen has it that Bodhidharma meditated for nine years straight, and this resulted in his arms and legs atrophying and eventually falling off. This is how the Japanese Daruma obtained its current form of a limbless head and torso. Daruma is revered in Japan as a symbol of focus, self-discipline and perseverance, but Westerners might consider whether sitting for extended periods of time is worth it. And while children and adolescents are unlikely to sit in front of a screen or with a screen in hand for nine years at a time, the cumulative time spent in such positions is worth our consideration and scrutiny; screen devices may, metaphorically, be creating a generation of Darumas who aren't losing their limbs but may be losing other aspects of development and self.

Unlike Darumic meditation and sitting in front of screen devices, the intrinsic value of socialising and play in real time noted above is that such activities often get young people up and moving. Sedentary behaviour is intimately linked with being immersed in screen activity and there is evidence that sedentary behaviour during childhood and adolescence may be associated with numerous adverse health outcomes.[15] In other words, and simply stated, more time being sedentary while engaging with screen devices is related to poorer health outcomes for children and adolescents. Specifically, more time spent on screens has been linked to poorer mental health while TV viewing and video gaming have been linked with poor or unfavourable behavioural outcomes.[16] Being active, conversely, has numerous benefits.

Yes, most people are well aware that physical activity is good for the body, but they may not be fully aware that it is also good for the minds of young and old alike. Being active reduces the risk of depressive symptoms in children and adolescents and has positive effects on affective and cognitive function and academic outcomes including memory, resilience,

[15] Chapur et al. (2020).

[16] Ibid.

executive function and overall school performance.[17] A major challenge for parents, caregivers and educators then, is ensuring that children and adolescents spend more time being active in a world that is becoming increasingly sedentary.

There is growing evidence that young people are becoming twenty-first-century Darumas and spending more and more time sitting and 'being' on screens and less time moving about and 'being' active with others. Studies range with regard to the amount of time young people spend on 'screen device sedentary activity'. Some studies suggest that screen time amounts to almost half of the after-school time in children and over half of after-school time in adolescents and that children were spending as much as six and a half hours a day and adolescents more than seven hours a day sitting in front of screens.[18] Given the ubiquitous nature of screens in schools and homes we believe those are very conservative numbers. Moreover, high levels of sedentary behaviour associated with less physical activity in childhood and adolescence are the norm in most parts of the world and worryingly those patterns of behaviour are often established by early childhood.[19] In Australia, where we are based, similar data has been collated and reported. The physical activity levels of Australian children and adolescents have diminished since the turn of the century and remain consistently low despite greater access to, and availability of, open spaces.[20] This is an important consideration given that the outdoors and natural environments not only offer a place to play and be active but also spaces that are healthy, potentially therapeutic and healing.

The Healing Power of Mother Nature

Have you ever considered hugging a tree? No, we're not talking about embracing a particular environmental perspective or gathering with activists to save the planet. We are literally wondering if you have ever

[17] Hillman et al. (2008); Voss et al. (2011); Erickson et al. (2019); Arida and Teixeira-Machado (2021).

[18] Kontostoli et al. (2021); See also, Pate et al. (2011); Arundell et al. (2016).

[19] Reilly et al. (2022).

[20] Hesketh et al. (2023); Australian Institute of Health and Welfare (AIHW) (2024).

hugged a tree and if you haven't, perhaps you should. You may find tree hugging therapeutic!

In 1984, an architecture, yes architecture not medicine or psychology, Professor by the name of Roger Ulrich published a rather curious set of findings. He studied the medical records of patients recovering from gall bladder surgery between 1972 and 1981 in a suburban Pennsylvania hospital. This cohort of patients was placed in a ward with rooms that had one of two views from their respective windows. One of the views afforded patients a natural setting with trees while other patients would stare out at a brick wall. Ulrich's findings were curious to say the least. Patients who looked out at trees got better quicker and with less intervention than those who were confined to a room facing bricks and mortar.[21]

The data from Ulrich's study were statistically significant and quite extraordinary. Those patients who could simply see trees from their rooms during recovery needed fewer, and less potent, drugs, had shorter postoperative days in hospital, had fewer complications and fewer negative evaluations in the nurse's notes. Notes from nurses regarding patients who looked at the brick wall included things such as patients being upset and crying or in need of a great deal of encouragement. Those who looked out at the greenery of trees and shared their thoughts with the nurses were found to be mostly positive, in good spirits and progressing well.

Another study by Ulrich is equally interesting and worth noting. Not satisfied with being able to see trees from a window, Ulrich and his colleagues explored whether similar benefits might be achieved by simply viewing pictures of landscapes.

In 1993, at Uppsala University Hospital in Sweden, Ulrich and his research team randomly assigned simulated window views of large nature photographs or abstract paintings to some of the one hundred and sixty heart surgery patients in the intensive care unit for viewing. The nature photographs included an open tree lined stream and a shadowy forest scene while the abstract paintings were of a white panel or blank wall. Some patients were not given anything to look at. Not too dissimilar to his earlier study, nature had a healing effect with those patients assigned the water and tree scene doing better than the other patients. They were

[21] Ulrich (1984).

less anxious and needed fewer doses of strong pain medicine than those who looked at the darker forest photograph, abstract art or no pictures at all.[22]

Taken in its entirety, Ulrich's work is rather astonishing. Two sets of surgery patients in two different countries had better postoperative surgical outcomes due to seeing nature through a window or as a large photograph. The strongest healing effects were the result of simply seeing trees so imagine what hugging one might do!

Since Ulrich published his first study, researchers from a wide range of disciplines have empirically demonstrated the healing power derived from being exposed to mother nature. We have a great deal of data telling us that contact with nature is linked to increases in a sense of wellbeing, positive emotions including happiness, positive social interactions, decreases in mental distress and a greater sense of meaning and purpose in life.[23]

Indeed, there is now plenty of evidence to highlight an innate and inherent need for living things to connect with other living things, and that artificial substitutes hold little value. For example, Attention Restoration Theory (ART) and Stress Recovery Theory (SRT) offer further platforms for understanding how nature appears to exert an array of healing properties.

ART was first coined by Rachel and Stephen Kaplan, and suggests that man-made objects (hard edges, geometric shapes) are more cognitively taxing to process compared to natural objects. In other words, the built environment is harder for us to process in our minds as our subconscious struggles with those things that are not natural. For example, next time you are in a dense urban environment, stop and consider how comfortable you feel immersed in concrete and steel with sharp angles, cold facades or bright neon lights. A conscious focus on such infrastructure can lead to cognitive overload and attention fatigue. However, our subconscious minds can also bring us to feeling tired from such elements without thinking of them by being simply immersed in those spaces. Fortunately, and according to ART, the opportunities to simply

[22] Ulrich et al. (1993).

[23] Bratman et al. (2019).

experience nature scenes and elements, especially water features through exposure to natural environments can help in diminishing such over-load and fatigue.[24] The term 'soft fascination' has been provided as a way of recognising that natural environments are not cognitively taxing to look at and provide opportunities for reflection, and a form of restorative practice for alleviating attention fatigue.[25]

SRT is not too dissimilar to ART but does tap into the field of evolutionary psychology by suggesting that human beings are biologically primed to feel better in natural, vegetation-rich environments.[26] Both ART and SRT have been supported by numerous other researchers and there is little doubt that being in nature has therapeutic benefits.[27] For those who are curious, a key question is what are the mechanisms behind mother nature's restorative properties? *Biophilia* is one hypothesis.

The word biophilia has its origins from the Greek words 'bios' meaning 'life' and 'philia' meaning 'love of' and literally means love of life or living things. It was popularised in the 1960s by the German-American social psychologist and psychoanalyst Erich Fromm and formerly used in his work entitled *The Anatomy of Human Destructiveness* where he described biophilia as a passionate love of life and all that is living.[28]

The term was later used by the American biologist and Emeritus Professor of Harvard, Edward O. Wilson in book, *Biophilia: The Human Bond with Other Species*.[29] In this Pulitzer Prize winning volume, Wilson used the word biophilia to describe the connection that humans have with nature, a connection that is, in part, genetic. Wilson believed that we have an innate drive to focus on and affiliate with nature and his work prompted researchers in a wide range of fields to explore this phenomenon.

Let us consider that idea a bit further before moving on. For Wilson and others biophilia is more than a simple love of nature and isn't reserved for those who like being outdoors. Biophilia is a human instinct that calls us to have connections with nature as a product of

---

[24] Kaplan and Kaplan (1989).

[25] Kaplan (1995).

[26] Ulrich (1983); Ulrich et al. (1991).

[27] Hartig et al. (2014); Ohly et al. (2016).

[28] Fromm (1973).

[29] Wilson (1986).

our evolution. Some have referred to this evolutionary affinity with nature conceptually as 'environment of evolutionary adaptedness'.[30] It is underpinned with a notion that the natural environment of our ancient past has played a part in shaping humanity and remains prominent even though our lived environments have changed drastically.

So, could it be that humans have a deeply ingrained love of nature, a love that is intuitive, instinctual and imprinted in our DNA? The healing powers uncovered by Ulrich might suggest that there is something to this idea. Moreover, could it also be that when we replace those connections with artificial pretenders via screen devices, we thwart innate biological needs? We believe there is some merit in such considerations. Our contention, based on the evidence presented here and the preceding chapters, suggests that living in our current built environments and playing in virtual worlds while replacing real human interactions with digital 'friends' has led to a range of dysfunctional mental processes in young people. Social psychologist, bestselling author and Professor of Ethical Leadership at New York University, Jonathon Haidt would likely agree.

Professor Haidt has meticulously laid out a detailed and compelling look at the rise of anxiety and depressive disorders in children and adolescents.[31] He argues that advances in technology have given rise to a 'phone-based' childhood that started to emerge between 2010 and 2015. He suggests that children born during that time and beyond have had their childhoods rewired resulting in four foundational harms: social deprivation, sleep deprivation, attention fragmentation and addiction. We have spoken of these harms in previous chapters, but we think Haidt may have missed something, and we would add another foundational harm, 'Nature Deficit Disorder'.[32] The reasons for bringing this to your attention extend beyond some of the aspects of play, healing and movement noted above. For many children and adolescents opportunities to experience any aspects of the natural

---

[30] Bennett (2018).

[31] Haidt (2024).

[32] The term Nature-Deficit Disorder was introduced by Richard Louv in his book, *Last Child in the Woods: Saving Our Children from Nature-Deficit Disorder.*

environment are limited or if available, sanitised. We believe this contributes to deficits of opportunities for experiencing the natural environment and tacitly gives credence and permission to young people for being on screens in place of being in nature. If you allow us a bit of leeway, we will draw all of this together before the chapter ends.

Reclaiming a Balance Through the *GREAT* Outdoors

Before we further explore the human condition linking wellbeing and mother nature and its capacity for buffering the impact of screen devices on developing minds we'd like to offer some pertinent background and contextual information. Let's start this by acknowledging that as humans grow older and begin to navigate their environments with increased sophistication, they often get a huge degree of satisfaction in feeling effective and in control of themselves in their surroundings. Think, for example, of the look on a child's face when they take their first steps and have begun to master the puzzle of moving freely about their environment. If that does resonate perhaps you recall seeing looks of satisfaction when a teenager gets their driver's licence and a new sense of freedom. For parents these are often not just a time of pride but also one of nervous energy. You see, most human beings also prefer to exercise free will in choosing activities that appeal to them and children doing so can make parents anxious at times. For a young child, the newfound freedom that comes with increased capacities to move also plays into a child's curiosity and desire to exercise their free will to open cupboards and drawers and grab things including the oven door or a bottle of bleach. For teens, being independent of parents and able to transport themselves to wherever and whatever their hearts desire is free will at its finest, at least in their eyes. Nerve wracking as these events may be for parents, feeling in control and exercising free will are two crucial factors in building psychological wellbeing and are referred to by psychologists as 'competence' and 'autonomy'. Importantly, further development of competence and autonomy is not only unavailable via a screen but also most positively nurtured in particular scenarios. We refer to the importance of play once again to help explain this further.

Earlier we laid out some groundwork for understanding the importance of play for healthy development. Relatedly, the kind of play experiences that help cultivate both competence and autonomy are found via moderately but genuinely challenging environments; environments where children can test their abilities in self-assessment, problem-solving, risk-taking, and adaptation in response to challenge and failure. These types of experiences are particularly crucial during critical or sensitive periods when the brain is most receptive to such opportunities.

As important as challenging experiences are for children, such experiences can sometimes be problematic for adults because with challenge, comes risk. Occasionally that risk can be traumatic (e.g., a broken limb, concussion). However, and contrary to popular belief, research has shown that the hyper-sanitised, risk-averse play culture that we increasingly see in school yards and parks may well be counterproductive in terms of developing competence and autonomy. Adult preoccupations with safety and the avoidance of harm are not really in the best interests of child development. Safe playgrounds, as perceived through parental eyes may offer less than those that allow for elements of risk.

When researchers involved in the Sydney Playground Project released children into a playground with 44-gallon drums, old milk cartons, ropes, old tyres and other certain death traps compared to children in more conventional and safe playgrounds they produced some interesting findings. Not only were the children in the 'less safe environment' more active and less sedentary than their safer counterparts, but there was also a reduction in fighting and bullying in those playgrounds with random objects and greater freedom.[33] Similar experiences in New Zealand support the findings in Sydney. This occurred when the principal of a primary school in Auckland decided to add a variable to a university study focused on encouraging active play in the school grounds by abandoning all playground rules. Some parts of the playground became a 'loose parts pit' with pieces of wood, old tyres and even an old fire hose to play with while in other areas children were permitted to engage in mudslides,

[33] Perkins (2014); see also Bundy et al. (2017).

skateboarding, tree climbing and other nontraditional activities. The end results saw less children getting hurt, more children involved in physical activity and fewer problem behaviours including bullying compared to past experiences in the 'safe' playground and other traditional safe play areas.[34] Both the Sydney and Auckland playground experiments left the parents, teachers and researchers somewhat dumbfounded and asking why? Why are less safe and less supervised playgrounds producing positive results and fewer problems than safer play areas? Autonomy and competence are strong factors in these results.

Children can and will learn to take responsibility for their own safety, and the safety of others, if adults let them. When we withhold, from our children, the autonomy to take risks, learn from failures, discover coping techniques that are adaptive and problem-focussed, we withhold opportunities to build competence and ***learn.*** In overly safe playgrounds designed by risk averse adults and monitored by similarly risk averse parents and teachers, children's growing brains fail to develop autonomy, competence, self-discipline, good decision-making, good self-assessment of ability, high failure tolerance, and a smorgasbord of other cognitive and psychological benefits. But wait, there's more!

In hyper-sanitising play experiences, adults "hardwire" children to become psychologically fragile, fearful, avoidant and helpless in the face of challenge and failure; rather than facilitating their opportunities to innovate, problem-solve, bounce back from failure and adapt as they go forth to meet life's inevitable challenges, adults coddle children into fragility. In their eagerness to protect against largely imagined non-threats, adults have counterproductively introduced a downstream raft of highly problematic outcomes for children and adolescents. We believe that these, and other concerns, over safety have played a significant role in increasing the amount of time children and adolescents spend at home and on their devices and there is some strong evidence to support that assertion.

Earlier in the chapter we referred to Professor Jonathon Haidt's work exploring the rise of anxiety and depressive disorders amongst children since 2012. We also mentioned that he believed that the increase in

[34] Hill (2014).

mental health issues is part of an ongoing phenomenon of 'rewiring' childhood. One factor we did not mention at that time was his theory on the rapid and very unhelpful rise of 'safetyism'. For Professor Haidt safetyism is a "culture or belief system in which safety has become a sacred value" and "safety trumps everything else, no matter how unlikely or trivial the potential danger".[35] In an earlier work, and in collaboration with author and journalist Greg Lukianoff, Professor Haidt explored safetyism in the context of psychological safety and trauma.[36] We feel that perceptions of safety are certainly a factor in parental decisions around how their children play, engage with nature and take risks. Perhaps being at home on a screen is a 'safer' alternative in the eyes of some parents. Screens at home offer an illusion of safety; children are in the safe environment of home and not in parks, the playground or on the streets where danger might be lurking around a corner. However, as we noted in Chap. 7, virtual worlds may be physically safer compared to falling off a swing or bicycle, but they can also be a playground for predators and an environment not entirely well-suited for a developing mind. It also seems odd to us that children and adolescents are increasingly spending less time meeting at the mall or hanging out at a park.

In her work examining the lives of 'iGen'ers', Jean Twenge, author and Professor of Psychology at San Diego University, meticulously dissects generational data and uncovers a precipitous decline in face-to-face interactions between young people beginning at the turn of the century. For Professor Twenge, iGen'ers are those born between 2007 and 2010 who have grown up with smartphones. Echoing the work of Professor Haidt, Twenge documents changes in behaviours and attitudes of young people leading them to becoming relentless homebodies, afraid to take risks, unlikely to meet with others and as a consequence grow up to be less happy and prepared for the 'real' world.[37]

In Australia, Planet Ark commissioned a report in 2011 and found that in one generation, Australian children went from 73% to 13% playing outside more than inside with only one in five of children ever having

[35] Haidt (2024, p. 89).
[36] Lukianoff and Haidt (2018).
[37] Twenge (2017).

climbed a tree.[38] Similar findings have been echoed across a range of studies and reports. For example, one study found that a significant proportion of Australian children spend less than 30 minutes a day playing outdoors after school and that much of the free-time historically used for being outside has been replaced by screen devices.[39] A range of evidence tells us that one out of two children world-wide spends less than an hour a day outside while we also know that maximum security prisoners in Australia, Canada and the United States are guaranteed two hours of outdoor time daily.[40]

We noted earlier the potential implications of deficits in time children spend playing but equally important are deficits in time spent outdoors. Some researchers have found that the chances of developing a psychiatric disorder *decreased* incrementally the longer children had been surrounded by green space from birth to age ten years.[41] Such evidence highlights the importance of access to 'nature play' during the brain's sensitive period of growth. Perhaps the question to consider now, is given the weight of evidence presented in this chapter, what are the key points and potential courses of action for those seeking optimal developmental opportunities for children and teens.

Create Buffers and Shift the Balance

We love movies! From *Aliens* to *Forest Gump* to *Spiderman*, going to a movie theatre, leaving our worlds behind and escaping into a cinematographic experience is generally a positive experience. Such positivity is sometimes lost when watching movies at home. We differ in age but movies at home, on our 'smart' TVs are now more commonplace and certainly more affordable. Annoyingly, it turns out that no matter how 'smart' a television is, its internal workings can be hostage to poor internet connectivity and 'buffering'. Speaking from experience,

[38] Planet Ark (2011).

[39] Wen et al. (2009); See also Royal Children's Hospital National Child Health Poll (2022).

[40] Burrows (2017); Martinko (2018); Queensland Corrective Services (2024).

[41] Engemann et al. (2019).

communications with technicians often end with them telling us that buffering results from a technical problem with the platform being used or from the internet service provider and in most cases buffering is a function of our internet speed. Not enough juice in the internet can mean watching the most annoying circuitous graphic spinning its virtual wheel. But buffering does give us pause to think or do something else if the opportunity is presented. This is what we are hoping you might do as we discuss how to buffer the potential issues associated with screen devices—pause and think and get the young people in your lives doing something else. We offer the following points as food for thought, and action!

Regardless of what you know about child and adolescent developmental research, you are likely intuitively aware of what is important for all aspects of development based on your own experiences or those of your parents and grandparents. We have offered some details throughout this book but in the end, there are some simple guidelines that will help ensure your children do not fall into a screen abyss of social media or any other of the virtual traps we have discussed.

First, and very simply, if your children have not been provided with a device due to their age or any other factor, don't give in to any pressure to do so. Be it from your children, their peers or the parents of peers who look to justify their decisions of giving devices to their own children, there isn't any real need for your child to have a smartphone, laptop or tablet until 16 years of age. Yes, you read that correctly, 16! We do acknowledge that in 2023 the United States Surgeon General, Vivek Murthy noted that young people under age 14 shouldn't use social media due to it contributing to young people's declining which he labelled as "the defining public mental health crisis of our time".[42] We share his concern but think his edict of 14 years does not go far enough. Remember the brain does not fully develop until we are in our 20s and that the teen years (all of them) are a time of neural refinement and reconstruction coupled with identity development and other important psychological parameters. Surely, and in context of human development, another two years without devices is not too much to ask when it comes to protecting

[42] Peetz (2023).

the developing brain and by association mental wellbeing. Therefore, if you are a new parent, one with small children or one that has simply, for whatever reason, not embraced screens for your children, avoid doing so. In this sense do not buffer but instead build a blockade!

We know that adopting the measures above may be challenging. There will be parents and teachers, among others, who will look to push and/or critique your parenting, but you are responsible for the wellbeing of your children not anyone else's nor are you responsible for any misguided societal norms or education 'mythinformation'. When a school looks to pressure you by insisting on the provision of a screen device, turn back to Chap. 3 and arm yourselves with the findings of the OECD or others who have questioned the educative value of screen engagement. After that, simply ask those in the school who oversee the curriculum or teaching to show you the empirical evidence supporting technology use as a mechanism for improved outcomes. Chances are they won't do so because such evidence is scant at best and scientifically disingenuous at its worst. And if they show you a government report, ignore it unless the report has numerous empirical studies in a reference list to support its claims. Too often government reports are premised on other government reports which are based on other government reports in a perpetual cycle of dubious evidence gathering. If asking for evidence doesn't seem to sway any decisions then perhaps remind them that both Bill Gates and the late Steve Jobs had very strict rules about screen use with their own children in the knowledge that time on screens was not in the best interests of their children's development.[43] Or if all else fails, have them read your copy of this book!

Second, if your children are fully immersed in using a device then work to wean them off slowly, especially the adolescents in your world. Remember the importance of autonomy and competence?! Children who have grown up digital may not respond well to edicts of going cold turkey, but there is a caveat to that that we will discuss later. For now, try to remember that disengaging with a virtual world will need some coaching, transition and most importantly modelling.

---

[43] Mancini (2023).

Children will watch and mimic the adults around them, especially their parents! Children see, children do was the catchline of a television commercial in Australia that depicted a number of scenes where adults were behaving badly in front of their children who in turn copied the behaviour they saw. The end of the commercial sees a man stop to help a lady who has dropped some groceries in the car park and the young boy accompanying him does not hesitate to also help. The message of the commercial was simple enough and an example of what psychologists have come to know as 'social learning theory'. The essence of this theory is that learning can occur through observation, imitation, and modelling and it is a useful reminder here; children will often, not always, but often copy the behaviour they observe. You can probably see where this is going but if not, again it is quite simple. If you want children and adolescents off their devices or at the very least moderating their consumption it would be helpful for them to see you doing so as well. Turning devices off at a set time, putting devices away at meals or at times of communal gathering, getting outside and engaging with the outdoors, exercising without technology, or anything else that does not really require a device are some examples of modelling healthy behaviour. Moreover, if you disengage you will find it easier to argue that they should as well. Telling kids to get off their devices does not usually end well when the adult giving that command is not prepared to do likewise.

Third, shift the balance! For those children who spend more time in a virtual world than the real one, create boundaries and shift that time. As noted above, being with others, play and physical activity are key factors for healthy development. It should also be clear that getting outside is good for us and nature serves as perhaps the best buffer to all the possible negative impacts of too much time on screens. This book has noted that there's an ever-growing body of research looking at screen time associated with various psychological disorders and autistic-like symptoms in particular. It also noted that an impressive set of interventions by clinicians was to simply remove children from the screens, get them outdoors and remove the 'autism' to get them functioning more 'normally'.

The terms autism, and normally, are presented above in inverted commas for a reason worth noting before exploring nature as a therapeutic intervention further. We have written widely on the topic of 'virtual autism' across several platforms and various print media. Inevitably there are some who fail to hear our message and instead engage in ad hominem attacks by accusing us of 'ableism'. For those unaware of the term 'ableism', it is a form of discrimination in favour of able-bodied people. In other words, there are those who would cast us as individuals who view those with clinically diagnosed autism as somehow lesser versions of humanity than non-autistic individuals. So just to be clear, we do not eschew any measure of human worth associated with autism or the lack-there-of and this holds true for any divergence recognised as disorders by psychologists and psychiatrists alike. What we are saying is that children and adolescents who spend too much time on screen devices are displaying behaviours that would not normally be seen in the absence of such devices. We can say this with a degree of certainty given the expansive research noting digital detoxes through nature have not only enhanced psychological wellbeing but also those manifestations of behaviours that are a product of living in a digital world. Genuine, clinically diagnosed autism, does not disappear by being outdoors!

Earlier in the chapter we discussed research around the healing power of mother nature and what appears to be an innate desire for being as close to nature as often as possible. We noted how spending time in nature is linked to improvements in mood, mental health and emotional wellbeing. Remote and biodiverse green spaces may be particularly helpful, but as we found in Chaps. 4 and 5, even urban parks and trees can lead to positive outcomes. This suggests that we need to get children playing outside, a lot!

We also discussed the importance of play and physical activity. In terms of play, it is significant to note that outdoor play might even hold the power to change the trajectory of brain development for the better. For example, children who live closer to a park, and have access to open green spaces show enhanced cognition, fewer behavioural problems, a lower risk of developing ADHD and enhanced emotional wellbeing.[44] Proximity to green spaces has also been shown to buffer stressful events and improve a child's capacity to self-regulate.[45]

[44] Amoly et al. (2014); Flouri et al. (2014); McCormick (2017).

[45] Taylor et al. (2002).

This is good news for those children and adolescents whose minds have been temporarily wired into a daydream like state of disassociation with reality through incessant consumption of pixelated images and activities on screens. It reminds us of the importance of creating and nurturing opportunities to help children stay connected to the real world, build genuine friendships with actual people, develop their imagination, and learn how to negotiate, adapt and overcome challenges. Preparing a child for adulthood within the biological cradle of nature and relationships ensures the best foundation to learn, overcome and succeed. Human beings find purpose and meaning in life and bolster their emotional states and social skills largely through the social and cultural context created by contact, in real time, with others.[46] In the end, buffering screen disorders in young people simply requires a commitment to get them off their screens and connecting with people in real time and in real environments. Not doing so casts them into an abyss of developmental uncertainty!

Summary

This final chapter consolidates how excessive screen time displaces critical developmental experiences for children and adolescents. Human beings are fundamentally social creatures whose brains and wellbeing depend on meaningful face-to-face interactions. Play—particularly self-directed and dramatic play—is essential for cognitive, social-emotional and physical development. Yet screen time has dramatically reduced both social interaction and active play, creating increasingly sedentary lifestyles with documented negative health outcomes.

The chapter highlights the therapeutic benefits of nature exposure, drawing on concepts like Attention Restoration Theory, Stress Recovery Theory, and biophilia to demonstrate how natural environments support mental health and cognitive functioning. Research shows that access to nature correlates with improved mental health outcomes,

[46] Kardaras (2016).

while time in challenging outdoor environments develops crucial competence and autonomy.

The authors argue that modern "safetyism" has contributed to children's increased screen dependence by limiting outdoor exploration. They recommend delaying device access until age 16, modelling healthy technology use, and creating boundaries that shift the balance towards real-world experiences, particularly in nature, to buffer against the negative impacts of excessive screen time on developing brains.

Bibliography and Further Reading

Amoly, E., Dadvand, P., Forns, J., Lopez-Vincente, M., Basagana, X., Julvez, J., Alvarez-Pederol, M., Nieuwenhuijsen, M.J. & Sunyer, J. (2014). Green and blue spaces and behavioral development in Barcelona schoolchildren: The BREATHE Project. *Environmental Health Perspectives*, 122(12), 1351–1358. https://doi.org/10.1289/ehp.1408215

Arida, R.M. & Teixeira-Machado, L. (2021). The contribution of physical exercise to brain resilience. *Frontiers in Behavioural Neuroscience*, 14:626769. https://doi.org/10.3389/fnbeh.2020.626769

Arundell L, Fletcher E, Salmon J, Veitch J & Hinkley T. (2016) A systematic review of the prevalence of sedentary behavior during the after-school period among children aged 5–18 years. *International Journal of Behavioral Nutrition and Physical Activity*, 13(1), 1–9. https://doi.org/10.1186/s12966-016-0419-1

Australian Institute of Health and Welfare (AIHW) (2024). Physical activity. https://www.aihw.gov.au/reports/physical-activity/physical-activity. Accessed August 28, 2024.

Barnett, W.S., Jung, K., Yarosz, D.J., Thomas, J., Hornbeck, A., Stechuk, R. & Burns, S. (2008). Educational effects of the Tools of the Mind curriculum: A randomized trial. *Early Childhood Research Quarterly*, 23(3), 299–313. https://doi.org/10.1016/j.ecresq.2008.03.001

Bennett, K. (2018). Environment of evolutionary adaptedness (EEA). In V. Zeigler-Hill, & T Shackelford (Eds) *Encyclopedia of Personality and Individual Differences* (pp.1–3). Springer.

Bjorklund, D.F., & Pellegrini, A.D. (2002). Homo Ludens: The importance of play. In D.F. Bjorklund & A.D. Pellegrini (Eds.), *The Origins of Human*

Nature: Evolutionary Developmental Psychology, (pp. 297–331). American Psychological Association

Bratman, G.N., Anderson, C.B., Berman, M.G., et al (2019). Nature and mental health: An ecosystem service perspective. *Science Advances*, 5(7), https://doi.org/10.1126/sciadvaax0903

Bundy, A., Engelen, L., Wyver, S., Tranter, P., Ragen, J., Bauman, A., Baur, L., Schiller, W., Simpson, J.M., Niehues, A.N., Perry, G., Jessup, G., & Naughton, G. (2017). Sydney Playground Project: A cluster randomized trial to increase physical activity, play and social skills. *Journal of School Health*, 87(10), 751–759. https://doi.org/10.1111/josh.12550

Burrows, S. (2017). We lock our kids up longer than we do maximum security convicts. *Newsweek*, October 27th. https://www.newsweek.com/we-lock-our-kids-longer-we-do-maximum-security-convicts-694845. Accessed September 12th, 2024.

Carson, V., Hunter, S., Kuzik, N., Gray, C.E., Poitras, V.J., Chaput, J., Saunders, T.J., Katzmarzyk, P.T., Okely, A.D., Gorber, S.C., Kho, M.E., Sampson, M., Lee, H. & Tremblay, M.S. (2016). Systematic review of sedentary behaviour and health indicators in school-aged children and youth: An update. *Applied Physiology, Nutrition, and Metabolism*, 41(6 Suppl 3), S240–265. https://doi.org/10.1139/apnm-2015-0630.

Carter, C. S. (2007). Neuropeptides and the protective effects of social bonds. In E. Harmon-Jones & P. Winkielman (Eds.), *Social Neuroscience: Integrating Biological and Psychological Explanations of Social Behavior* (pp. 425–438). The Guilford Press.

Chapur, J., Willumsen, J., Bull, F., Chou, R., Ekelund, U. Firth, J., Jago, R., Ortega, F.B. & Katzmarzyk, P.T. (2020). 2020 WHO guidelines on physical activity and sedentary behaviour for children and adolescents aged 5–17 years: Summary of evidence. *International Journal of Behavioral Nutrition and Physical Activity*, 17(141). https://doi.org/10.1186/s12966-020-01037-z

Christiansen, J., Qualter, P., Friss, K., Pedersen, S.S., Lund, R., Andersen, C.M., Bekker-Jeppsesen, M. & Lasgaard, M. (2021). Associations of loneliness and social isolation with physical and mental health among adolescents and young adults. *Perspectives in Public Health*, 141(4), 226–236. https://doi.org/10.1177/17579139211016077

Cloud, D.H., Drucker, E., Browne, A. & Parsons, J. (2015) Public health and solitary confinement in the United States. *American Journal of Public Health*, 105(1), 18–26. https://doi.org/10.2105/AJPH.2014.30220

Cozolino, L. (2013). *The Social Neuroscience of Education: Optimizing Attachment & Learning in the Classroom*. W.W. Norton & Company.

Diamond, A., Barnett, W.S., Thomas, J. & Munro, S. (2007). Preschool program improves cognitive control. *Science*, 318(5855), 1387–1388. https://doi.org/10.1126/science.1151148

Elkind, D. (2007). *The Power of Play: Learning What Comes Naturally*. Da Capo Lifelong Books.

Engemann, K., Pederson, C.B., Arge, L., Tsirogiannis, C., Mortenson, P.B. & Svenning, J.C. (2019). Residential green space in childhood is associated with lower risk of psychiatric disorders from adolescence into adulthood. *Proceedings of the National Academy of Sciences*, 116(11), 5188–5193. https://doi.org/10.1073/pnas.1807504116

Erickson, K.I., Hillman, C., Stillman, C.M., Ballard, R.M., Bloodgood, B., Conroy, D.E., Macko, R., Marquez, D.X., Petruzzello, S.J. & Powell, K.E. (2019). Physical activity, cognition, and brain outcomes: A review of the 2018 physical activity guidelines. *Medicine & Science in Sports & Exercise*, 51(6), 1242–1251. https://doi.org/10.1249/MSS.0000000000001936

Flouri, E., Midouhas, E. & Joshi, H. (2014). The role of urban neighbourhood green space in children's emotional and behavioural resilience. *Journal of Environmental Psychology*, 40, 179–186. https://doi.org/10.1016/j.jenvp.2014.06.007

Fromm, E.S. (1973). *The Anatomy of Human Destructiveness*. Holt, Reinhart & Winston.

Haidt, J. (2024). *The Anxious Generation: How the Great Rewiring of Childhood is Causing an Epidemic of Mental Illness*. Allen Lane.

Hartig, T., Mitchell, R., de Vries, S., & Frumkin, H. (2014). Nature and health. *Annual Review of Public Health, 35*(1), 207–228. https://doi.org/10.1146/annurev-publhealth-032013-182443.

Hesketh, D., Booth, V., Cleland, V., Gomersall, S.R., Olds, T., Reece, L., Ridgers, N.D., Straker, L., Stylianou, M., Tomkinson, G.R. (2023). Results from the Australian 2022 Report Card on physical activity for children and young people. *Journal of Exercise Science & Fitness*, 21(1), 83–87. https://doi.org/10.1016/j.jesf.2022.10.006

Hill, M. (2014). School ditches rules and loses bullies. *Stuff – Digital News Provider*. https://www.stuff.co.nz/national/education/9650581/School-ditches-rules-and-loses-bullies Accessed September 5th, 2025.

Hillman, C.H., Erickson, K.I. & Kramer, A.F. (2008). Be smart, exercise your heart: Exercise effects on brain and cognition. *Nature Review Neuroscience*, 9, 58–65. https://doi.org/10.1038/nrn2298

Johnston, O., Wildy, H. & Shand, J. (2023). Teenagers learn through play too: Communicating high expectations through a playful learning approach. *Australian Educational Research.* 50, 921–940. https://doi.org/10.1007/s13384-022-00534-3

Kaplan, S. (1995). The restorative benefits of nature: Toward an integrative framework. *Journal of Environmental Psychology*, 15(3), 169–182. https://doi.org/10.1016/0272-4944(95)90001-2

Kaplan, R. & Kaplan, S. (1989). *The Experience of Nature: A Psychological Perspective.* Cambridge University Press.

Kardaras, N. (2016). *Glow Kids: How Screen Addiction is Hijacking Our Kids – And How to Break the Trance.* St. Martin's Griffin.

Kontostoli, E., Jones, A.P., Pearson, N., Foley, L., Biddle, S.J.H. & Atkin, A.J. (2021). Age-related change in sedentary behavior during childhood and adolescence: A systematic review and meta-analysis.

Lockwood, R. & Connor, S. (2017). Playfulness in adults: An examination of play and playfulness and their implications for coaching. *Coaching: An International Journal of Theory, Research and Practice*, 10(1), 54–65. https://doi.org/10.1080/17521882.2016.1268636

Lukianoff, G. & Haidt, J. (2018). *The Coddling of the American Mind: How Good Intentions and Bad Ideas Are Setting Up a Generation For Failure.* Penguin Press.

Mancini, J. (2023). Hidden side of Steve Jobs and Bill Gates: The banned their kids from iPads and other devices they created. *Yahoo!Finance*, August 12th, 2023. https://finance.yahoo.com/news/hidden-side-steve-jobs-bill-165424007.html Accessed September 17th, 2024.

Martinko, K. (2018). Children spend less time outside than prison inmates. *Treehugger*, October 11th, 2018. https://www.treehugger.com/children-spend-less-time-outside-prison-inmates-4857353 Accessed September 12th, 2024.

Maslow, A. (1970). *Religions, Values, and Peak-Experiences.* Viking.

Maslow, A. (1999). Toward a Psychology of Being – 3rd Edition. John Wiley & Sons

McCormick, R. (2017). Does access to green space impact the mental well-being of children: A systematic review. *Journal of Pediatric Nursing*, 37, 3–7. https://doi.org/10.1016/j.pedn.2017.08.027

Medina, J. (2010). *Brain Rules for Baby: How to Raise a Smart and Happy Child from Zero to Five.* Pear Press.

Nagel, M. C. (2012). *In The Beginning: The Brain, Early Development and Learning.* Australian Council for Educational Research (ACER).

Ohly, H., White, M.P., Wheeler, B.W., Bethel, A., Ukoumunne, O.C., Nikolaou, V., & Garside, R. (2016). Attention Restoration Theory: A systematic review of the attention restoration potential of exposure to natural environments. *Journal of Toxicology and Environmental Health*. Part B, Critical reviews, 19(7), 305–343. https://doi.org/10.1080/10937404.2016.1196155.

Pancani, L., Marinucci, M., Aureli, N. & Riva, P. (2021). Forced social isolation and mental health: A study on 1,006 Italians under COVID-19 lockdown. *Frontiers in Psychology*, 12:663799. https://doi.org/10.3389/fpsyg.2021.663799

Panksepp, J. (2004). *Affective Neuroscience: The Foundations of Human and Animal Emotions*. Oxford University Press.

Panksepp, J. & Biven, L. (2012). *The Archaeology of Mind: Neuroevolutionary Origins of Human Emotion*. W. W. Norton & Company.

Pate, R.R., Mitchell, J.A., Byun, W. & Dowda, M. (2011). Sedentary behaviour in youth. *British Journal of Sports Medicine*, 45(11), 906–913. https://doi.org/10.1136/bjsports-2011-090192

Pavin Ivanec, T. (2022). The lack of academic social interactions and students' learning difficulties during COVID-19 faculty lockdowns in Croatia: The mediating role of the perceived sense of life disruption caused by the pandemic and the adjustment to online studying. *Social Sciences*, 11(2), 42. https://doi.org/10.3390/socsci11020042

Peetz, C. (2023). Kid's declining mental health is the 'crisis of our time', Surgeon General says. *Education Week*, April 25th. https://www.edweek.org/leadership/kids-declining-mental-health-is-the-crisis-of-our-time-surgeon-general-says/2023/04. Accessed September 19th, 2024.

Pellegrini, A.D., Dupuis, D. & Smith, P.K. (2007). Play in evolution and development. *Developmental Review*, 27(2), 261–276. https://doi.org/10.1016/j.dr.2006.09.001

Perkins, M. (2014). Over-protected, over-organised…why kids need time to play. *Sydney Morning Hearld*, July 17th. https://www.smh.com.au/technology/overprotected-overorganised%2D%2Dwhy-kids-need-time-to-play-20140716-ztq7p.html Accessed September 5th, 2024.

Pietrabissa, G. & Simpson, S.G. (2020). Psychological consequences of social isolation during COVID-19 outbreak. *Frontiers in Psychology*, 11:2201. https://doi.org/10.2289/fpsyg.2020.02201

Planet Ark (2011). *Climbing Trees: Getting Aussie Kids Back Outdoors*. https://treeday.planetark.org/documents/doc-534-climbing-trees-research-report-2011-07-13-final.pdf Accessed September 9th, 2024.

Porges, S.W. (2003). Social engagement and attachment: A phylogenetic perspective. *Annals of the New York Academy of Sciences, 1008*, 31–47.

Queensland Corrective Services (2024). *Prisoner Accommodation Management ACC: Maximum Security Unit – Custodial Operations Practice Directive.* www.publications.qld.gov.au/ckan-publications-attachments-prod/resources/2ab478b9-82db-4e04-a093-9ca69ddbf93e/maximum-security-unit-copd-redacted.pdf?ETag=080f396c5e0154026497da73ce4c881a. Accessed September 12th, 2024.

Reilly, J.J., Barnes, J., Gonzales, S., Huang, W.Y., Manyanga, T., Tanaka, C. & Tremblay, M.S. (2022). Recent secular trends in child and adolescent physical activity and sedentary behaviour internationally: Analyses of Active Healthy Kids Global Alliance global matrices 1.0 to 4.0. *Journal of Physical Activity and Health*, 19, 729–736. https://doi.org/10.1123/jpah.2022-0312

Reiter, K., Ventura, J., Lovell, D., Augustine, D., Barragan, M., Blair, T, Chesnut, K., Dashtgard, P., Gonzales, G., Pifer, N. & Strong, J. (2020). Psychological distress in solitary confinement: Symptoms, severity, and prevalence in the United States, 2017–2018. *American Journal of Public Health*, 110(S1), 556–562. https://doi.org/10.2105/AJPH.2019.305375

Royal Children's Hospital National Child Health Poll (2022). *Australian Families: How We Play – Poll Number 28.* Royal Children's Hospital Melbourne.

Sapolsky, R.M. (2017). *Behave: The Biology of Humans At Our Best and Worst.* Penguin Press.

Smith, P.K. (1982). Does play matter? Functional and evolutionary aspects of animal and human play. *Behavioral and Brain Sciences*, 5(1), 139–184. https://doi.org/10.1017/S0140525X0001092X

Taylor, A.F., Kuo, F.E. & Sullivan, W.C. (2002). Views of nature and self-discipline: Evidence from inner city children. *Journal of Environmental Psychology*, 22(1–2), 49–63. https://doi.org/10.1006/jevp.2001.0241

Twenge, J.M. (2017). *iGen: Why Today's Super-Connected Kids Are Growing Up Less Rebellious, More Tolerant, Less Happy – and Completely Unprepared for Adulthood.* Atria Books.

Ulrich, R.S. (1983). Aesthetic and affective response to natural environment. In I. Altman, & J.F. Wohlwill (Eds). *Human Behavior and Environment – Volume 6* (pp. 85–125). Plenum Press.

Ulrich, R.S. (1984). View through a window may influence recovery from surgery. *Science*, 224(4647), 420–421. https://doi.org/10.1126/science.6143402.

Ulrich, R.S., Simons, R.F., Losito, B.D., Fiorito, E., Miles, M.A., & Zelson, M. (1991). Stress recovery during exposure to natural and urban environments. *Journal of Environmental Psychology*, 11(3), 201–230. https://doi.org/10.1016/S0272-4944(05)80184-7

Ulrich, R.S., Lunden, O. & Eltinge, J.L. (1993). Effects of exposure to nature and abstract pictures on patients recovering from open heart surgery. *Society for Psychophysiological Research (U.S.) Meeting 33*, S7.

Voss, M.W., Nagamatsu, L.S., Liu-Ambrose, T. & Kramer, A.F. (2011). Exercise, brain, and cognition across the life span. *Journal of Applied Physiology*, 111(5), 1505–1513. https://doi.org/10.1152/japplphysiol.00210.2011

Wen, L.M., Kite, J., Merom, D. & Rissel, C. (2009). Time spent playing outdoors after school and its relationship with independent mobility: A cross-sectional survey of children aged 10–12 years in Sydney, Australia. *International Journal of Behavioral Nutrition and Physical Activity*, 6(15). https://doi.org/10.1186/1479-5868-6-15

Wilson, E.O. (1986). *Biophilia: The Human Bond With Other Species*. Harvard University Press.

Epilogue

Like slow-to-learn children, we keep repeating the mistakes of the past and forgetting a fundamental lesson from history that keeps repeating itself: humanity's most ambitious inventions and technological advances are inseparable from their dark side. From Icarus to Oppenheimer, taking a bite from the fruit of the tree of knowledge comes at a steep price. Dr Nicholas Kardaras[1]

When we set out to write this book we were fully aware that there would be critics accusing us of being Luddites and out of touch with reality. We are also aware that there are plenty of individuals and organisations, including big tech and social media companies, who might debunk all we have discussed. Indeed, there is no shortage of proponents of screen use who suggest that screens and social media offer support and a potential lifeline for troubled youth. As altruistic as that sounds, most, if not all, of those people have vested interests in ensuring screens are part and parcel of growing up digital. Motives are always important to consider so here are ours.

[1] Kardaras (2022, p. 186).

M. C. Nagel, R. Sharman, *Virtual Autism and Other Screen Disorders*, Palgrave Studies in Cyberpsychology, https://doi.org/10.1007/978-3-032-00803-9

We work in the areas of child and adolescent development and psychology and have carved our careers out of doing so. We are also parents with some of our children on the cusp of having their own children and others still in the early stages of childhood so we think that affords us some practical insights to couple with our research and scholarly activities. We don't claim to be 'the experts' in all the content we have provided but we do think we have a substantive degree of experience and expertise that gives us some latitude to present cogent and hopefully thought-provoking arguments. At the core of those arguments is an underlying concern that with limited scrutiny and an overzealous embracing of screens and screen devices we have taken a bite from the fruit of the tree of knowledge that now appears to be enacting a steep and as yet not well understood price.

Bibliography and Further Reading

Abbott, A. (2013). Solving the brain. *Nature Neuroscience*, volume 499 (July 18), 272–273.

American Psychiatric Association (2013). *Diagnostic and Statistical Manual of Mental Disorders (DSM-5) – 5th Edition.* American Psychiatric Association Publishing.

Amoly, E., Dadvand, P., Forns, J., Lopez-Vincente, M., Basagana, X., Julvez, J., Alvarez-Pederol, M., Nieuwenhuijsen, M.J. & Sunyer, J. (2014). Green and blue spaces and behavioral development in Barcelona schoolchildren: The BREATHE Project. *Environmental Health Perspectives*, 122(12), 1351–1358. https://doi.org/10.1289/ehp.1408215

Arida, R.M. & Teixeira-Machado, L. (2021). The contribution of physical exercise to brain resilience. *Frontiers in Behavioural Neuroscience*, 14:626769. https://doi.org/10.3389/fnbeh.2020.626769

Arnett, J.J. (1999). Adolescent storm and stress, reconsidered. *American Psychologist*, 54(5), 317–326. https://doi.org/10.1037/0003-066X.54.5.317

Arundell L, Fletcher E, Salmon J, Veitch J & Hinkley T. (2016) A systematic review of the prevalence of sedentary behavior during the after-school period among children aged 5–18 years. *International Journal of Behavioral Nutrition and Physical Activity*, 13(1), 1–9. https://doi.org/10.1186/s12966-016-0419-1

M. C. Nagel, R. Sharman, *Virtual Autism and Other Screen Disorders*, Palgrave Studies in Cyberpsychology, https://doi.org/10.1007/978-3-032-00803-9

Australian Institute of Health and Welfare (AIHW) (2024). Physical activity. https://www.aihw.gov.au/reports/physical-activity/physical-activity. Accessed August 28, 2024.

Baio et al. (2018). Prevalence of Autism Spectrum Disorder Among Children Aged 8 Years - Autism and Developmental Disabilities Monitoring Network, 11 Sites, United States, 2014. *Morbidity and Mortality Weekly Report – Surveillance Summaries*; Washington, D.C. 2018 Apr 27;67(6):1–23. https://doi.org/10.15585/mmwr.ss6706a1

Bahia, V.S., Takada, L.T., Caixeta, L., Lucato, L.T., Porto, C.S. & Nitrini, R. (2013). Prefrontal damage in childhood and changes in the development of personality: A case report. *Dementia Neuropsychologia*, 7(1), 132–135. https://doi.org/10.1590/S1980-57642013DN70100019

Bandura, A. (1962). *Social Learning Through Imitation*. University of Nebraska Press.

Bandura, A. (1977). *Social Learning Theory*. Prentice Hall.

Bandura, A., & Walters, R.H. (1963). *Social Learning and Personality Development*. Holt, Rinehart & Winston Inc.

Barker, F.G. (1995). Phineas among the phrenologists: The American crowbar case and nineteenth-century theories of cerebral localization. *Journal of Neurosurgery*, 82(4), 672–682. https://doi.org/10.3171/jns.1995.82.4.0672

Barnett, W.S., Jung, K., Yarosz, D.J., Thomas, J., Hornbeck, A., Stechuk, R. & Burns, S. (2008). Educational effects of the Tools of the Mind curriculum: A randomized trial. *Early Childhood Research Quarterly*, 23(3), 299–313. https://doi.org/10.1016/j.ecresq.2008.03.001

Bennett, K. (2018). Environment of evolutionary adaptedness (EEA). In V. Zeigler-Hill, & T Shackelford (Eds) *Encyclopedia of Personality and Individual Differences* (pp.1–3). Springer.

Blakemore, S.J. (2008). The social brain in adolescence. *Nature Reviews Neuroscience*, 9(4), 267–277. https://doi.org/10.1038/nm2353/

Bjorklund, D.F., & Pellegrini, A.D. (2002). Homo Ludens: The importance of play. In D.F. Bjorklund & A.D. Pellegrini (Eds.), *The Origins of Human Nature: Evolutionary Developmental Psychology*, (pp. 297–331). American Psychological Association

Borst J.P., Taatgen, N. A. & van Rijn, H. (2010). The problem state: a cognitive bottleneck in multitasking. *Journal of Experimental Psychology, Learning, Memory and Cognition*, 36(2), 363–82. https://doi.org/10.1037/a0018106. PMID: 20192536.

Bratman, G.N., Anderson, C.B., Berman, M.G., et al (2019). Nature and mental health: An ecosystem service perspective. *Science Advances*, 5(7), https://doi.org/10.1126/sciadvaax0903

Brockmyer, J.F. (2014). Video games. In V.C. Strasburger, B.J. Wilson & A.B Jordan (Eds.), *Children, Adolescents and the Media – Third Edition*, (pp. 457–486). Sage.

Browne, K.D. & Hamilton-Giachristsis, C. (2005). The influence of violent media on children and adolescents: A public-health approach. *The Lancet*, 365(9460), 702–710. https://doi.org/10.1016/S0140-6736(05)17952-5

Brüne, M. & Brüne-Cohrs, U. (2006). Theory of mind – evolution, ontogeny, brain mechanisms and psychopathology. *Neuroscience and Biobehavioral Reviews*, 30(4), 437–455. https://doi.org/10.1016/j.neubiorev.2005.08.001.

Broyd, J., Boniface, L., Parsons, D., Murphy, D. & Hafferty, J.D. (2023). Incels, violence and mental disorder: A narrative review with recommendations for best practice in risk assessment and clinical intervention. *BJPsych Advances*, 29, 254–264. https://doi.org/10.1192/bja.2022.15

Bryson, B. (2019). *The Body: The Guide for Occupants.* Doubleday.

Buchholz, K. (2019). How much of the internet consists of porn? *Statista*, February 11th. https://www.statista.com/chart/16959/share-of-the-internet-that-is-porn/#:~:text=Only%204%20percent%20of%20websites,might%20bring%20about%20new%20insights. Accessed January 25th, 2025.

Bundy, A., Engelen, L., Wyver, S., Tranter, P., Ragen, J., Bauman, A., Baur, L., Schiller, W., Simpson, J.M., Niehues, A.N., Perry, G., Jessup, G., & Naughton, G. (2017). Sydney Playground Project: A cluster randomized trial to increase physical activity, play and social skills. *Journal of School Health*, 87(10), 751–759. https://doi.org/10.1111/josh.12550

Burrows, S. (2017). We lock our kids up longer than we do maximum security convicts. *Newsweek*, October 27th. https://www.newsweek.com/we-lock-our-kids-longer-we-do-maximum-security-convicts-694845. Accessed September 12th, 2024.

Carson, V., Hunter, S., Kuzik, N., Gray, C.E., Poitras, V.J., Chaput, J., Saunders, T.J., Katzmarzyk, P.T., Okely, A.D., Gorber, S.C., Kho, M.E., Sampson, M., Lee, H. & Tremblay, M.S. (2016). Systematic review of sedentary behaviour and health indicators in school-aged children and youth: An update. *Applied Physiology, Nutrition, and Metabolism*, 41(6 Suppl 3), S240–265. https://doi.org/10.1139/apnm-2015-0630.

Carter, C. S. (2007). Neuropeptides and the protective effects of social bonds. In E. Harmon-Jones & P. Winkielman (Eds.), *Social Neuroscience: Integrating*

Biological and Psychological Explanations of Social Behavior (pp. 425–438). The Guilford Press.

Carter, R. (2009). *The Human Brain Book: An Illustrated Guide To Its Structure, Function and Disorders.* D.K. Publishing.

Casey, B.J., Somerville, L.H., Gotlib, I.H., Ayduk, O., Franklin, N.T., Askren, M.K., Jonides, J., Berman, M.G., Wilson, N.L., Teslovich, T., Glover, G., Zayas, V., Mischel, W. & Shoda, Y. (2011). Behavioral and neural correlates of delay gratification 40 years later. *Proceedings of the National Academy of Sciences*, 108(36), 14998–15003. https://doi.org/10.1073/pnas.1108561108

Chabris, C. & Simons, D. (2010). *The Invisible Gorilla: And Other Ways Our Intuitions Deceive Us.* Harmony.

Chapur, J., Willumsen, J., Bull, F., Chou, R., Ekelund, U. Firth, J., Jago, R., Ortega, F.B. & Katzmarzyk, P.T. (2020). 2020 WHO guidelines on physical activity and sedentary behaviour for children and adolescents aged 5–17 years: Summary of evidence. *International Journal of Behavioral Nutrition and Physical Activity*, 17(141). https://doi.org/10.1186/s12966-020-01037-z

Christiansen, J., Qualter, P., Friss, K., Pedersen, S.S., Lund, R., Andersen, C.M., Bekker-Jeppsesen, M. & Lasgaard, M. (2021). Associations of loneliness and social isolation with physical and mental health among adolescents and young adults. *Perspectives in Public Health*, 141(4), 226–236. https://doi.org/10.1177/17579139211016077

Cloud, D.H., Drucker, E., Browne, A. & Parsons, J. (2015) Public health and solitary confinement in the United States. *American Journal of Public Health*, 105(1), 18–26. https://doi.org/10.2105/AJPH.2014.30220

Collini, S. (2010). *That's Offensive: Criticism, Identity, Respect.* Seagull Books.

Corlett, D. & Crabbe, M. (2013). *Love and Sex in an Age of Pornography* (Streamed online). Retrieved from https://www.kanopy.com/en/usc/product/love-and-sex-age-pornography

Cozolino, L. (2013). *The Social Neuroscience of Education: Optimizing Attachment & Learning in the Classroom.* W.W. Norton & Company.

Crugnola, C.R., Tambelli, R., Spinelli, M., Gazzoti, S., Caprin, C. & Albizzati, A. (2011). Attachment patterns and emotion regulation strategies in the second year. *Infant Behaviour & Development*, 34(1), 136–151. https://doi.org/10.1016/j.inbeh.2010.11.002

Cuzzolin, F., Morelli, A., Cîrstea, B. & Sahakian, B.J. (2020). Knowing me, Knowing you: Theory of Mind in AI. *Psychological Medicine*, 50, 1057–1061. https://doi.org/10.1017/S0033291720000835.

D'angelo, E. (2019). The cerebellum gets social. *Science*, 363(6424), 229. https://doi.org/10.1126/science.aaw2571.

Dadvand et al (2018). The association between lifelong greenspace exposure and 3-dimensional brain magnetic resonance imaging in Barcelona schoolchildren. *Environmental Health Perspectives*, 126(2). https://doi.org/10.1289/EHP1876

Dahl, R.E. (2004). Adolescent brain development: A period of vulnerabilities or opportunities. *Annals of the New York Academy of Sciences*, 1021, 1–22. https://doi.org/10.1196/annals.1308.001

Diamond, A., Barnett, W.S., Thomas, J. & Munro, S. (2007). Preschool program improves cognitive control. *Science*, 318(5855), 1387–1388. https://doi.org/10.1126/science.1151148

Dong, H.Y., Feng, J.Y, Wang, B., Shan, L. & Jia, F.Y. (2021) Screen Time and Autism: Current Situation and Risk Factors for Screen Time among Pre-School Children with ASD. *Frontiers in* Psychiatry, 12:675902. https://doi.org/10.3389/fpsyt.2021.675902

Donovan, G.H., Michael, Y.L., Gatziolis, D., Mannetje, A, & Douwes, J. (2019). Association between exposure to the natural environment, rurality, and attention-deficit hyperactivity disorder in children in New Zealand: A linkage study. *The Lancet: Planetary Health*, 3(5), E226–E234. https://doi.org/10.1016/S2542-5196(19)30070-1

Durston, S., Davidson, M.C., Tottenham, N., Galvan, A., Spicer, J., Fossella, J.A. & Casey, B.J. (2006). A shift from diffuse to focal cortical activity with development. *Developmental Science*, 9(1), 1–8. https://doi.org/10.1111/j.1467-7687.2005.00454.x

Eagleman, D. (2020). *Livewired: The Inside Story of the Ever-Changing Brain.* Pantheon Books, New York.

El-Hamamsy, D., Parmar, C., Shoop-Worrall, S., & Reid, F.M. (2022). Public understanding of female genital anatomy and pelvic organ prolapse (POP); a questionnaire-based pilot study. *International Urogynecology Journal, 33*(2), 309–318. https://doi.org/10.1007/s00192-021-04727-9.

Elkind, D. (2007). *The Power of Play: Learning What Comes Naturally.* Da Capo Lifelong Books.

Engemann, K., Pederson, C.B., Arge, L., Tsirogiannis, C., Mortenson, P.B. & Svenning, J.C. (2019). Residential green space in childhood is associated with lower risk of psychiatric disorders from adolescence into adulthood. *Proceedings of the National Academy of Sciences*, 116(11), 5188–5193. https://doi.org/10.1073/pnas.1807504116

Erickson, K.I., Hillman, C., Stillman, C.M., Ballard, R.M., Bloodgood, B., Conroy, D.E., Macko, R., Marquez, D.X., Petruzzello, S.J. & Powell, K.E. (2019). Physical activity, cognition, and brain outcomes: A review of the 2018 physical activity guidelines. *Medicine & Science in Sports & Exercise*, 51(6), 1242–1251. https://doi.org/10.1249/MSS.0000000000001936

Erikson, E.H. (1950). *Childhood and Society*. Norton.

Erikson, E.H. (1959). Identity and the life cycle. *Psychological Issues*, 1, 1–171.

Erikson, E.H. (1968). *Identity, Youth and Crisis*. Norton.

Fikkers, K.M., Piotrowski, J.T., Lugtig, P. & Valkenburg, P.M. (2016). The role of perceived peer norms in the relationship between media violence exposure and adolescents' aggression. *Media Psychology*, 19(1), 4–26. https://doi.org/10.1080/15213269.2015.1037960

Filippi, R., Ceccolini, A., Periche-Tomas, E. & Bright, P. (2020). Developmental trajectories of metacognitive processing and executive function from childhood to older age. *Quarterly Journal of Experimental Psychology*, 73(11), 1757–1773. https://doi.org/10.1177/1747021820931096

Fitzsimmons, C. (2023). Frances Haugen blew the whistle on Facebook two years ago. This is what happened next. The Sydney Morning Herald, October 9, 2023.

Foulkes, L. (2021). *Losing Our Minds: The Challenge of Defining Mental Illness*. St Martin's Press.

Flouri, E., Midouhas, E. & Joshi, H. (2014). The role of urban neighbourhood green space in children's emotional and behavioural resilience. *Journal of Environmental Psychology*, 40, 179–186. https://doi.org/10.1016/j.jenvp.2014.06.007

Fried, C. B. (2008). In-class laptop use and its effects on student learning. *Computers & Education*, 50(3), 906–914.

Fromm, E.S. (1973). *The Anatomy of Human Destructiveness*. Holt, Reinhart & Winston.

Giedd, J. (2001). *Frontline: Inside the teenage brain – An interview with Professor Jay Giedd*. Television documentary. Arlington Virginia: Public Broadcasting Service.

Giedd, J.N. (2004). Structural magnetic resonance imaging of the adolescent brain. *Annals of the New York Academy of Sciences, 1021*(1), 77–85. https://doi.org/10.1196/annals.1308.009

Giedd, J.N., Vaituzis, C., Hamburger, S. D., Lange, N., Rajapakse, J. C., Kaysen, D., Vauss, Y. C., & Rapoport, J. L. (1996). Quantitative MRI of the temporal lobe, amygdala and hippocampus in normal human development:

Ages 4–18 years. *Journal of Comparative Neurology, 366*(2), 223–230. https://doi.org/10.1002/(SICI)1096-9861(19960304)366:2<223::AID-CNE3>3.0.CO;2-7

Goldberg, E. (2001). *The Executive Brain: Frontal Lobes and the Civilized Mind.* Oxford University Press, Oxford, UK.

Goleman, D. (1995). *Emotional Intelligence: Why It Can Matter More Than IQ.* Bantam Books.

Graham, P. (2023). Transgender children and young people: How the evidence can point a way forward. *BJPsyche Bulletin*, 47(2), 98–104. https://doi.org/10.1192/bjb.2022.3

Grossman, M. (2023). *Lost in Trans Nation: A Child Psychiatrists Guide Out of the Madness*. Skyhorse Publishing.

Haidt, J. (2024). *The Anxious Generation: How the Great Rewiring of Childhood is Causing an Epidemic of Mental Illness.* Allen Lane.

Hall, G. (1904). *Adolescence: Its Psychology and Its Relations to Physiology, Anthropology, Sociology, Sex, Crime, Religion and Education (Volumes I & II).* Prentice-Hall.

Harle, B. (2019) Intensive early screen exposure as a causal factor for symptoms of autistic spectrum disorder: The case for Virtual autism. *Trends in Neuroscience and Education*, 17, 100119. https://doi.org/10.1016/j.tine.2019.100119

Hartig, T., Mitchell, R., de Vries, S., & Frumkin, H. (2014). Nature and health. *Annual Review of Public Health, 35*(1), 207–228. https://doi.org/10.1146/annurev-publhealth-032013-182443.

Hatfield, E., Cacioppo, J.T. & Rapson, R.L. (1994). *Emotional Contagion: Studies in Emotions & Social Interaction*. Cambridge University Press.

Hattie, J. (2013). *Visible Learning and the Science of How We Learn.* Routledge, London.

Hayes, B. &Bainton, J. (2020) The impact of reduced sleep on school related outcomes for typically developing children aged 11–19: A systematic review. *School Psychology International,* 41(6), 569–594. https://doi.org/10.1177/0143034320961130

Heffler K.F., Sienko D.M., Subedi K., McCann K.A., Bennett D. S. (2020) Association of early-life social and digital media experiences with development of autism spectrum disorder–like symptoms. *JAMA Pediatrics* 174(7):690–696. https://doi.org/10.1001/jamapediatrics.2020.0230

Hesketh, D., Booth, V., Cleland, V., Gomersall, S.R., Olds, T., Reece, L., Ridgers, N.D., Straker, L., Stylianou, M., Tomkinson, G.R. (2023). Results from the Australian 2022 Report Card on physical activity for children and young people. *Journal of Exercise Science & Fitness*, 21(1), 83–87. https://doi.org/10.1016/j.jesf.2022.10.006

Higley, J.D. (1995). Primates in alcohol research. *Alcohol Health Research World*, 19(3), 213–216. PMCID: PMC6875760 PMID:31798031

Hill, M. (2014). School ditches rules and loses bullies. *Stuff – Digital News Provider.* https://www.stuff.co.nz/national/education/9650581/School-ditches-rules-and-loses-bullies Accessed September 5th, 2025.

Hillman, C.H., Erickson, K.I. & Kramer, A.F. (2008). Be smart, exercise your heart: Exercise effects on brain and cognition. *Nature Review Neuroscience*, 9, 58–65. https://doi.org/10.1038/nrn2298

Hoffer, E. (1955). *The Passionate State of Mind, and Other Aphorisms*. Harper.

Horvath, M., Alys, L., Massey, K., Pina, A., Scally, M., & Adler, J.R. (2013). *Basically...porn is everywhere. A Rapid Evidence Assessment on the Effects that Access and Exposure to Pornography has on Children and Young People*. Office of the Children's Commissioner.

Hu, S., Tucker, L., Wu, C. & Yang, L. (2020). Beneficial effects of exercise on depression and anxiety during the Covid-19 pandemic: A narrative review. *Frontiers in Psychiatry*, 11:587557. https://doi.org/10.3389/fpsyt.2020.587557

Hu, W., Hao, Z., Du, P., Di Vincenzo, F., Manzi, G., Cui, J., Fu, Y., Pan, Y. & Li, H. (2023).Genomic inference of a severe human bottleneck during the Early to Middle Pleistocene transition. *Science,* 381(6661), 979–984. https://doi.org/10.1126/science.abq7487

Hubel, D.H. & Wiesel, T.N. (1970). The period of susceptibility to the physiological effects of unilateral eye closure in kittens. *Journal of Physiology*, 206, 419–436.

Hutton, J.S., Dudley, J., Horowitz-Kraus, T., DeWitt, T. & Holland, S.K. (2020). Associations between screen-based media use and brain white matter integrity in preschool-aged children. *JAMA Pediatrics*, 174(1), e193869. https://doi.org/10.1001/jamapediatrics.2019.3869.

Hutton, J.S., Dudley, J., DeWitt, T. & Horowitz-Kraus, T. (2022). Associations between digital media use and brain surface structural measures in preschool-aged children. *Scientific Reports*, 12, 19095. https://doi.org/10.1038/s41598-022-20922-0

Jack, B. (2014). Goethe's *Werther* and its effects. *The Lancet Psychiatry*, 1(1), 18–19. https://doi.org/10.1016/S2215-0366(14)70229-9

Jacobs, A. (2017). *How to Think: A Survival Guide for a World at Odds.* Crown Publishing Group.

Jammel, M. (2024). Death grip syndrome – What is it and reverse technique. *Fortius Health Clinic for Happy Healthy Live*, 27th November. Available at https://www.fortiushealthclinic.com/blog/death-grip-syndrome-what-is-it-and-reverse-technique (Accessed 14th April, 2025).

Johnson, Z. (2013). Fifty shades of grey release date pushed back to February 13, 2015 – Just in time for Valentine's Day. *ENews*, 13th November. Available at https://www.eonline.com/news/480515/fifty-shades-of-grey-release-date-pushed-back-to-february-13-2015-just-in-time-for-valentine-s-day (Accessed 17th January, 2025).

Johnston, O., Wildy, H. & Shand, J. (2023). Teenagers learn through play too: Communicating high expectations through a playful learning approach. *Australian Educational Research.* 50, 921–940. https://doi.org/10.1007/s13384-022-00534-3

Kakabadse, A.P., Kakabadse, N.K., Bailey, S. & Myers, A. (2009). *Techno Addicts: Young Person Addiction to Technology,* Sigel Press.

Kaplan, S. (1995). The restorative benefits of nature: Toward an integrative framework. *Journal of Environmental Psychology*, 15(3), 169–182. https://doi.org/10.1016/0272-4944(95)90001-2

Kaplan, R. & Kaplan, S. (1989). *The Experience of Nature: A Psychological Perspective.* Cambridge University Press.

Kardaras, N. (2016). *Glow Kids: How Screen Addiction is Hijacking Our Kids – And How to Break the Trance.* St. Martin's Griffin.

Kardaras, N. (2022). *Digital Madness: How Social Media is Driving Our Mental Health Crisis and How to Restore Our Sanity.* St. Martin's Press.

Khan, A., Lee, E. Y., Rosenbaum, S., Khan, S. R., & Tremblay, M. S. (2021). Dose-dependent and joint associations between screen time, physical activity, and mental wellbeing in adolescents: an international observational study. *The Lancet. Child & Adolescent Health*, *5*(10), 729–738. https://doi.org/10.1016/S2352-4642(21)00200-5

Kernberg, O.F., & Caligor, E. (2005). A psychoanalytic theory of personality disorders. In M.F. Lenzenweger, & J. Clarkin (Eds.), *Major Theories of Personality Disorders* (2nd ed.). The Guilford Press.

Klimstra, T. & van Doeselaar, L. (2017). Identity formation in adolescence and young adulthood. In j. Specht (Ed.), *Personality Development Across the Lifespan*, Chapter 18, pp. 293–308. Academic Press. *Obesity Reviews*, 22(9), e13263. https://doi.org/10.1111/0br.13263

Kontostoli, E., Jones, A.P., Pearson, N., Foley, L., Biddle, S.J.H. & Atkin, A.J. (2021). Age-related change in sedentary behavior during childhood and adolescence: A systematic review and meta-analysis.

Korones, S. (2012). Ethiopian kids teach themselves using only tablet computers. www.zdnet.com/article/ethiopian-kids-teach-themselves-using-only-tablet-computers.

Kushima et al., (2022). Association between screen time exposure in children at 1 year of age and autism spectrum disorder at 3 years of age The Japan Environment and Children's Study. JAMA Pediatrics, 176(4), 384–391. https://doi.org/10.1001/jamapediatrics.2021.5578

LeDoux, J. (1998). *The Emotional Brain: The Mysterious Underpinnings of Emotional Life.* Simon & Schuster Inc, New York.

Linning, S. (2014). Is your child's new iPad a magnet for paedophiles? Ten-year-old girl groomed through tablet by perverts despite her parents taking 'all sensible safety measures', UK Daily Mail, 27th December. Available at https://www.dailymail.co.uk/news/article-2888300/Is-child-s-new-iPad-magnet-paedophiles-Ten-year-old-girl-groomed-tablet-perverts-despite-parents-taking-sensible-safety-measures.html (Accessed 1st May, 2024).

Lockwood, R. & Connor, S. (2017). Playfulness in adults: An examination of play and playfulness and their implications for coaching. *Coaching: An International Journal of Theory, Research and Practice*, 10(1), 54–65. https://doi.org/10.1080/17521882.2016.1268636

Louie, D.W. (2017). Social media and the sexual exploitation of Indigenous girls. *Girlhood Studies*, 10(2), 97–113. https://doi.org/10.3167/ghs.2017.100208

Louv, R. (2008) *Last Child in the Woods: Saving Our Children from Nature-Deficit Disorder.* Algonquin Books.

Lukianoff, G. & Haidt, J. (2018). *The Coddling of the American Mind: How Good Intentions and Bad Ideas Are Setting Up a Generation For Failure.* Penguin Press.

MacLean, P.D. (1990). *The Triune Brain in Evolution: Role in Paleocerebral Functions.* Springer.

MacMillan, M. (2002). *An Odd Kind of Fame. Stories of Phineas Gage.* MIT Press.

Mancini, J. (2023). Hidden side of Steve Jobs and Bill Gates: The banned their kids from iPads and other devices they created. *Yahoo!Finance*, August 12th, 2023. https://finance.yahoo.com/news/hidden-side-steve-jobs-bill-165424007.html Accessed September 17th, 2024.

Marengo, D., Longobardi, C., Fabris, M.A., & Settanni, M. (2018). Highly-visual social media and internalizing symptoms in adolescence: The mediating role of body image concerns. *Computers in Human Behavior, 82*, 63–69. https://doi.org/10.1016/j.chb.2018.01.003.

Marques, P. Madeira, T. & Gama, A. (2022). Menstrual cycle among adolescents: Girl's awareness and influence of age at menarche and overweight. *Revista Paulista de Pediatria*, Jan 5, 40:e2020494. https://doi.org/10.1590/1984-0462/2022/40/2020494

Marston, C., & Lewis, R. (2014). Anal heterosex among young people and implications for health promotion: A qualitative study in the UK. *BMJ Open, 4*(8), e004996. https://doi.org/10.1136/bmjopen-2014-004996.

Martinko, K. (2018). Children spend less time outside than prison inmates. *Treehugger*, October 11th, 2018. https://www.treehugger.com/children-spend-less-time-outside-prison-inmates-4857353 Accessed September 12th, 2024.

Maslow, A. (1970). *Religions, Values, and Peak-Experiences*. Viking.

Maslow, A. (1999). Toward a Psychology of Being – 3rd Edition. John Wiley & Sons

Masten, A.S., Hubbard, J.J., Gest, S.D., Tellegen, A., Garmezy, N. & Ramirez, M. (1999). Competence in the context of adversity: Pathways to resilience and maladaptation from childhood to late adolescence. *Development and Psychopathology,* 11 (1), 143–169. https://doi.org/10.1017/s0954579499001996

Masten, C.L., Telzer, E.H., Fuligni, A.J., Lieberman, M.D. & Eisenberger, N.I. (2012). Time spent with friends in adolescence relates to less neural sensitivity to later peer rejection. *Social Cognitive and Affective Neuroscience*, 7(1), 106–114. https://doi.org/10.1093/scan/nsq098

Mathews, V.P., Kronenberger, W.G., Wany, Y., Lurito, J.T., Lowe, M.J. & Dunn, D.W. (2005). Media violence exposure and frontal lobe activation measured by functional magnetic resonance imaging in aggressive and non-aggressive adolescents. *Journal Of Computer Assisted Tomography*, 29(3), 287–292. https://doi.org/10.1097/01.rct0000162822.46958.33

Maza, M.T., Fox, K.A. & Kwon, S. (2023). Association of habitual checking behaviours on social media with longitudinal functional brain development. *JAMA Pediatrics*, 177(2), 160167. https://doi.org/10.1001/jamapediatrics.2022.4924.

McCormick, R. (2017). Does access to green space impact the mental well-being of children: A systematic review. *Journal of Pediatric Nursing*, 37, 3–7. https://doi.org/10.1016/j.pedn.2017.08.027

McNicol, M.L., & Thorsteinsson, E.B. (2017). Internet addiction, psychological distress, and coping responses among adolescents and adults. *Cyberpsychology, Behavior and Social Networking, 20*(5), 296–304. https://doi.org/10.1089/cyber.2016.0669.

Medina, J. (2010). *Brain Rules for Baby: How to Raise a Smart and Happy Child from Zero to Five.* Pear Press.

Meinhardt-Injac, B., Dau, M.M. & Meinhardt, G. (2020). Theory of mind development from adolescence to adulthood: Testing the two-component model. *British Journal of Developmental Psychology*, 38(2), 289–303. https://doi.org/10.1111/bjdp.12320.

Miller, G.A. (1956). The magical number seven, plus or minus two: some limits on our capacity for processing information, *Psychological Review*, 63(2), 81–97. https://doi.org/10.1037/h0043158

Mischel, W. (2014). *The Marshmallow Test: Understanding Self-Control and How to Master It.* Bantam Press.

Mischel, W. & Ebbesen, E.B. (1970). Attention in the delay of gratification. *Journal of Personality and Social Psychology*, 16(2), 329–337. https://doi.org/10.1037/h0029815

Mischel, W., Ebbesen, E.B. & Raskoff Zeiss, A. (1972). Cognitive and attentional mechanisms in delay of gratification. *Journal of Personality and Social Psychology*, 21(2), 204–218. https://doi.org/10.1037/h0032198

Mitchell, K. J. (2018). *Innate: How the Wiring of Our Brains Shapes Who We Are.* Princeton University Press.

Mitchell, K.J., Finkelhor, D., & Wolak, J. (2003). The exposure of youth to unwanted sexual material on the internet: A national survey of risk, impact, and prevention. *Youth & Society, 34*(3), 330–358. https://doi.org/10.1177/0044118X02250123 (Original work published 2003).

Mitra, S., Dangwal, R., Chatterjee, S., Jha, S., Bisht, R.S. & Kapur, P. (2005). Acquisition of computer literacy on shared public computers: Children and the 'hole in the wall'. Australasian Journal of Educational Technology, 21(3), 407–426. https://doi.org/10.14742/ajet.1328

Moreno, M. & Kota, R. (2014). Social media. In V.C. Strasburger, B.J. Wilson & A.B Jordan (Eds.), *Children, Adolescents and the Media – Third Edition*, (pp. 435–456). Sage.

Mrug, S., Madan, A. & Windle, M. (2015). Emotional desensitization to violence contributes to adolescents' violent behaviour. *Journal of Abnormal Child Psychology*, 44, 75–86. https://doi.org/10.1007/s10802-015-9986-x

Murray, J.P. (2012). Children and media violence: Behavioural and neurological effects of viewing violence. In W. Warburton & D. Braunstein (Eds.), Growing Up Fast and Furious (pp. 34–55). The Federation Press.

Nagel, M. C. (2012). *In The Beginning: The Brain, Early Development and Learning.* Australian Council for Educational Research (ACER).

Nagel, M.C. (2014). *In the Middle: The Adolescent Brain, Behaviour and Learning.* Australian Council for Educational Research (ACER).

Nagel, M.C. (2019). Neurobiology of risk taking and impulsivity. In M. Nagel & R Sharman (Eds.), *The Encyclopedia of Child and Adolescent Development, Vol 8 – Biology, Neurology and Cognition in Adolescence* (pp. 1–8). Wiley-Blackwell Publishing Ltd. https://doi.org/10.1002/9781119171492.wecad361

Nagel, M.C. (2021). *It's A Girl Thing: Understanding the Neuroscience Behind Educating and Raising Girls.* Amba Press.

Nagel, M. C., & Scholes, L. (2016). Understanding Development and Learning: Implications for Teaching. Oxford University Press.

Newbury, C.R., Crowley, R., Rastle, K. & Tamminen, J. (2021). Sleep deprivation and memory: Meta-analytic reviews of studies on sleep deprivation before and after learning. *Psychological Bulletin*, 147(11), 1215–1240. https://doi.org/10.1037/bul0000348.

Nguyen, H.B., Loughead, J., Lipner, E., Hantsoo, L., Kornfield, S.L. & Epperson, C.N. (2019). What has sex got to do with it? The role of hormones in the transgender brain. *Neuropsychopharmacology*, 44(1), 22–37. https://doi.org/10.1038/s41386-018-0140-7

Ogas, O. & Gaddam, S. (2012). *A Billion Wicked Thoughts: What the Internet Tells Us About Sexual Relationships.* Plume.

Ohly, H., White, M.P., Wheeler, B.W., Bethel, A., Ukoumunne, O.C., Nikolaou, V., & Garside, R. (2016). Attention Restoration Theory: A systematic review of the attention restoration potential of exposure to natural environments. *Journal of Toxicology and Environmental Health.* Part B, Critical reviews, 19(7), 305–343. https://doi.org/10.1080/10937404.2016.1196155.

Organisation For Economic Cooperation and Development (OECD) (2015). *Students, Computers and Learning: Making the Connection.* OECD Publishing, Paris, France. https://doi.org/10.1787/9789264239555-en

OECD (2023). *PISA 2022 Results (Volume I): The State of Learning and Equity in Education*, PISA, OECD Publishing. https://doi.org/10.1787/53f23881-en.

Oz, A. (2001).Big Ideas ABC Television. https://www.abc.net.au/radionational/programs/archived/radioeye/how-to-cure-a-fanatic%2D%2D-amos-oz/3475244#transcript

Pancani, L., Marinucci, M., Aureli, N. & Riva, P. (2021). Forced social isolation and mental health: A study on 1,006 Italians under COVID-19 lockdown. *Frontiers in Psychology*, 12:663799. https://doi.org/10.3389/fpsyg.2021.663799

Panksepp, J. (2004). *Affective Neuroscience: The Foundations of Human and Animal Emotions*. Oxford University Press.

Panksepp, J. (2014). Integrating bottom-up internalist views of emotional feelings with top-down externalist views: Might brain affective changes constitute reward and punishment effects within animal brains? *Cortex*, 59, 208–213. https://doi.org/10.1016/j.cortex.2014.04.15

Panksepp, J. & Biven, L. (2012). *The Archaeology of Mind: Neuroevolutionary Origins of Human Emotion*. W. W. Norton & Company.

Pate, R.R., Mitchell, J.A., Byun, W. & Dowda, M. (2011). Sedentary behaviour in youth. *British Journal of Sports Medicine*, 45(11), 906–913. https://doi.org/10.1136/bjsports-2011-090192

Pavin Ivanec, T. (2022). The lack of academic social interactions and students' learning difficulties during COVID-19 faculty lockdowns in Croatia: The mediating role of the perceived sense of life disruption caused by the pandemic and the adjustment to online studying. *Social Sciences*, 11(2), 42. https://doi.org/10.3390/socsci11020042

Peetz, C. (2023). Kid's declining mental health is the 'crisis of our time', Surgeon General says. *Education Week*, April 25th. https://www.edweek.org/leadership/kids-declining-mental-health-is-the-crisis-of-our-time-surgeon-general-says/2023/04. Accessed September 19th, 2024.

Pellegrini, A.D., Dupuis, D. & Smith, P.K. (2007). Play in evolution and development. *Developmental Review*, 27(2), 261–276. https://doi.org/10.1016/j.dr.2006.09.001

Perkins, M. (2014). Over-protected, over-organised…why kids need time to play. *Sydney Morning Hearld*, July 17th. https://www.smh.com.au/technology/overprotected-overorganised%2D%2Dwhy-kids-need-time-to-play-20140716-ztq7p.html Accessed September 5th, 2024.

Phillips, D.P. (1974). The influence of suggestion on suicide: Substantive and theoretical implications of the Werther Effect. *American Sociological Review*, 39(3), 340–354. https://doi.org/10.2307/2094294

Pietrabissa, G. & Simpson, S.G. (2020). Psychological consequences of social isolation during COVID-19 outbreak. *Frontiers in Psychology*, 11:2201. https://doi.org/10.2289/fpsyg.2020.02201

Pinker, S. (2009). *How the Mind Works.* W.W. Norton & Company.

Planet Ark (2011). *Climbing Trees: Getting Aussie Kids Back Outdoors.* https://treeday.planetark.org/documents/doc-534-climbing-trees-research-report-2011-07-13-final.pdf Accessed September 9th, 2024.

Porges, S.W. (2003). Social engagement and attachment: A phylogenetic perspective. *Annals of the New York Academy of Sciences, 1008*, 31–47.

Queensland Corrective Services (2024). *Prisoner Accommodation Management ACC: Maximum Security Unit – Custodial Operations Practice Directive.* www.publications.qld.gov.au/ckan-publications-attachments-prod/resources/2ab478b9-82db-4e04-a093-9ca69ddbf93e/maximum-security-unit-copd-redacted.pdf?ETag=080f396c5e0154026497da73ce4c881a. Accessed September 12th, 2024.

Reilly, J.J., Barnes, J., Gonzales, S., Huang, W.Y., Manyanga, T., Tanaka, C. & Tremblay, M.S. (2022). Recent secular trends in child and adolescent physical activity and sedentary behaviour internationally: Analyses of Active Healthy Kids Global Alliance global matrices 1.0 to 4.0. *Journal of Physical Activity and Health*, 19, 729–736. https://doi.org/10.1123/jpah.2022-0312

Reiter, K., Ventura, J., Lovell, D., Augustine, D., Barragan, M., Blair, T, Chesnut, K., Dashtgard, P., Gonzales, G., Pifer, N. & Strong, J. (2020). Psychological distress in solitary confinement: Symptoms, severity, and prevalence in the United States, 2017–2018. *American Journal of Public Health*, 110(S1), 556–562. https://doi.org/10.2105/AJPH.2019.305375

Riggio, R.E. & Riggio, C.R. (2023). Social Contagion in H.S. Friedman & C.H. Markey (Eds.), *Encyclopedia of Mental Health – 3rd Edition* (Vol 3, pp. 270–273). Elsevier. https://doi.org/10.1016/B978-0-323-91497-0.00192-2

Robinson, T.N., Banda, J.A., Hale, L., Lu, A.S., Fleming-Milici, F., Calvert, S.L. & Wartella, E. (2017). Screen media exposure and obesity in children and adolescence. *Pediatrics*, 140 (Suppl2), S97–S101. https://doi.org/10.1542/peds.2016-1758K

Royal Children's Hospital National Child Health Poll (2022). *Australian Families: How We Play – Poll Number 28.* Royal Children's Hospital Melbourne.

Ruder, D. B. (2008). A work in progress: The teen brain. *Harvard Review,* 3(1), 8–10.

Saad, G. (2020). *The Parasitic Mind: How Infectious Ideas Are Killing Common Sense.* Regnery Publishing.

Sadeghi, S., Pouretemad, H.R., Khosrowabadi, R., Fathabadi, J. & Nikbakht, S. (2021). Parent–child interaction effects on autism symptoms and EEG relative power in young children with excessive screen-time, Early Child Development and Care, 191(6), 827–836. https://doi.org/10.1080/03004430.2019.1649256

Sapolsky, R.M. (2017). *Behave: The Biology of Humans At Our Best and Worst.* Penguin Press.

Schaub, M. (2017). E.L. James has a new 'Fifty Shades": Darker from Christian's point of view. *Los Angeles Times,* 10th October. Available at https://www.latimes.com/books/jacketcopy/la-et-jc-fifty-shades-darker-20171010-story.html (Accessed 17th January, 2025).

Schawbel, D. (2012). Daniel Goleman on the importance of ecological intelligence. *Forbes,* 1st August. Available at https://www.forbes.com/sites/danschawbel/2012/08/01/daniel-goleman-on-the-importance-of-ecological-intelligence/ (Accessed 23rd April, 2025).

Schulz, S. & McDonald, S. (2024). 'Not my boy'. When teachers are harassed by students, some schools and parents fail to help. *The Conversation,* 21st August. Available at https://theconversation.com/not-my-boy-when-teachers-are-harassed-by-students-some-schools-and-parents-fail-to-help-237122 (Accessed 14th April, 2025).

Sebastian, C.L., Fontaine, N.M.G., Bird, G., Blakemore, S.J., De Brito, S.A., McCrory, E.J.P. & Viding, E. (2012). Neural processing associated with cognitive and affective Theory of Mind in adolescents and adults. *Social Cognitive and Affective Neuroscience,* 7(1), 53–63. https://doi.org/10.1093/scan/nsr023.

Shamay-Tsoory, S.G., Harari, H., Aharon-Peretz, J. & Levkovitz, Y. (2010). The role of the orbitofrontal cortex in affective theory of mind deficits in criminal offenders with psychopathic tendencies. *Cortex,* 46(5), 668–677. https://doi.org/10.1016/j.cortex.2009.04.008.

Sharman, R., Allen, A., van Niekerk, K., Coles, A., Manocha, R. & Foran, T. (2024). "What is normal?": A qualitative exploration of health practitioners reports of treating patients presenting with unpleasant sexual experiences. *Archives of Sexual Behaviour*, 53(10), 4099–4116. https://doi.org/10.1007/s10508-024-02994-3

Sigman, A. (2009). Well connected?: The biological implications of 'social networking'. *The Biologist*, 56(1), 14–20.

Sina, E., Buck, C., Veidebaum, T. et al (2021). Media use trajectories and risk of metabolic syndrome in European children and adolescents: The IDEFICS/I. Family cohort. *International Journal of Behavioral Nutrition and Physical Activity*, 18(134). https://doi.org/10.1186/s12966-021-01186-9

Slobodin, O., Heffler, K.F. & Davidovitch, M. (2019). Screen media and autism spectrum disorder: A systematic literature review. *Journal of Developmental & Behavioral Pediatrics* 40(4), 303–311. https://doi.org/10.1097/DBP.0000000000000654

Smith, P.K. (1982). Does play matter? Functional and evolutionary aspects of animal and human play. *Behavioral and Brain Sciences*, 5(1), 139–184. https://doi.org/10.1017/S0140525X0001092X

Steinberg, L., Dahl, R., Keating, D., Kupfer, D.J., Masten, A.S. & Pine, D.S. (2006). The study of developmental psychopathology in adolescence: Integrating affective neuroscience with the study of context. In D Cicchetti & D.J. Cohen, (Eds.), *Developmental Psychopathology, Vol 2: Developmental Neuroscience,* 2nd Ed., (pp. 710–741). John Wiley & Sons Inc.

Sullivan, L.E. (2009). *The SAGE Glossary of the Social and Behavioral Sciences.* SAGE Publications Inc.

Sweeney, M. S. (2009). *Brain, The Complete Guide: How It Develops, How It Works and How To Keep It Sharp.* National Geographic Society, Washington, D.C.

Sylwester, R. (2007). *The Adolescent Brain: Reaching for Autonomy.* Corwin Press.

Taylor, A.F., Kuo, F.E. & Sullivan, W.C. (2002). Views of nature and self-discipline: Evidence from inner city children. *Journal of Environmental Psychology*, 22(1–2), 49–63. https://doi.org/10.1006/jevp.2001.0241

Taylor, A.F. & Kuo, F.E. (2009). Children with attention deficits concentrate better after walk in the park. *Journal of Attention Disorders*, 12(5), 402–409. https://doi.org/10.1177/1087054708323000

Teles, R.V. (2020). Phineas Gage's great Legacy. *Dementia & Neuropsychologia*, 14(4), 419–421. https://doi.org/10.1590/1980-57642020dn14-040013

Thomas, G., Bennie, J.A., DeCocker, K., Castro, O. & Biddle, S.J.H. (2019). A descriptive epidemiology of screen-based devices by children and adolescents: A scoping review of 130 surveillance studies since 2000. *Child Indicators Research*, 13(3), 935–950. https://doi.org/10.1007/s12187-019-09663-1

Tombu, M.N., Asplund, C.L., Dux, P.E., Godwin, D., Martin, J.W. & Marois, R. (2011). A Unified attentional bottleneck in the human brain. *Proceedings of the National Academy of Sciences*, 108(33), 13426–13431. https://doi.org/10.1073/pnas.1103583108

Triandis, H.C. (1989). The self and social behaviour in differing cultural contexts. Psychological Review, 96(3), 506–520. https://doi.org/10.1037/0033-295X.96.3.506

Twenge, J.M. (2011). Generational differences in mental health: Are children and adolescents suffering more or less? *American Journal of Orthopsychiatry*, 81(4), 469–472. https://doi.org/10.1111/j.1939-0025.2011.01115.x

Twenge, J.M. (2017). *iGen: Why Today's Super-Connected Kids Are Growing Up Less Rebellious, More Tolerant, Less Happy – and Completely Unprepared for Adulthood.* Atria Books.

Twenge, J.M. & Campbell, W.K. (2013). *The Narcissism Epidemic: Living in the Age of Entitlement.* Atria Paperback.

Twenge, J.M., Joiner, T.E., Rogers, M.L., & Martin, G.N. (2018). Increases in depressive symptoms, suicide-related outcomes, and suicide rates among U.S. adolescents after 2010 and links to increased new media screen time. *Clinical Psychological Science, 6*(1), 3–17. https://doi.org/10.1177/2167702617723376.

Ulrich, R.S. (1983). Aesthetic and affective response to natural environment. In I. Altman, & J.F. Wohlwill (Eds). *Human Behavior and Environment – Volume 6* (pp. 85–125). Plenum Press.

Ulrich, R.S. (1984). View through a window may influence recovery from surgery. *Science*, 224(4647), 420–421. https://doi.org/10.1126/science.6143402.

Ulrich, R.S., Simons, R.F., Losito, B.D., Fiorito, E., Miles, M.A., & Zelson, M. (1991). Stress recovery during exposure to natural and urban environments. *Journal of Environmental Psychology*, 11(3), 201–230. https://doi.org/10.1016/S0272-4944(05)80184-7

Ulrich, R.S., Lunden, O. & Eltinge, J.L. (1993). Effects of exposure to nature and abstract pictures on patients recovering from open heart surgery. *Society for Psychophysiological Research (U.S.) Meeting 33*, S7.

Uhls, Y.T., Michikyan, M., Morris, J., Garcia, D., Small, G. W., Zgourou, E., & Greenfield, P. M. (2014). Five days at outdoor education camp without screens improves preteen skills with nonverbal emotion cues. *Computers and Human Behavior, 39*, 387–392.

Vannucci, A., Flannery, K.M., & Ohannessian, C.M. (2017). Social media use and anxiety in emerging adults. *Journal of Affective Disorders, 207*, 163–166. https://doi.org/10.1016/j.jad.2016.08.040

Voss, M.W., Nagamatsu, L.S., Liu-Ambrose, T. & Kramer, A.F. (2011). Exercise, brain, and cognition across the life span. *Journal of Applied Physiology*, 111(5), 1505–1513. https://doi.org/10.1152/japplphysiol.00210.2011

Voss, P., Thomas, M. E., Cisneros-Franco, J. M. & de Villers-Sidani, E. (2017). Dynamic brains and the changing rules of neuroplasticity: Implications for learning and recovery. *Frontiers in Psychology*, 8:1657.

Wang, Y., Mathews, V.P., Kalnin, A.J., Mosier, K.M., Dunn, D.W., Saykin, A.J. & Kronenberger, W.G. (2009). Short term exposure to violent video game induces changes in frontolimbic circuitry in adolescents. *Brain Imaging and Behaviour*, 3, 38–50. https://doi.org/10.1007/s11682-008-9058-8

Weaver, M., Allen, A. & Sharman, R. (Under review). Facets of unpleasant sexual experiences for heterosexual men. *Journal of Sex Research*.

Weimer, A.A., Parault Dowds, S.J., Fabricius, W.V., Schwanenflugel, P.J., & Suh, G.W. (2017). Development of constructivist theory of mind from middle childhood to early adulthood and its relation to social cognition and behavior. *Journal of Experimental Child Psychology, 154*, 28–45. https://doi.org/10.1016/j.jecp.2016.10.002.

Wen, L.M., Kite, J., Merom, D. & Rissel, C. (2009). Time spent playing outdoors after school and its relationship with independent mobility: A cross-sectional survey of children aged 10–12 years in Sydney, Australia. *International Journal of Behavioral Nutrition and Physical Activity*, 6(15). https://doi.org/10.1186/1479-5868-6-15

Wilson, E.O. (1986). *Biophilia: The Human Bond With Other Species*. Harvard University Press.

World Health Organisation (2024). *Hooking the Next Generation: How the Tobacco Industry Captures Young Customers*. World Health Organisation, Geneva.

Wilbrecht, L. (2018). Your twelve-year-old isn't just sprouting new hair but is also forming (and being formed by) new neural connections. In D. J. Linden (Ed.), *Think Tank: Forty Neuroscientists Explore the Roots of Human Experience* (pp. 45–51). Yale University Press.

Wood, E., Zivcakova, L., Gentile, P., Archer, K., De Pasquale, D. & Nosk, A. (2011). Examining the impact of off-task multi-tasking with technology on real-time classroom learning. *Computers & Education*, 58(1), 365–374.

Yang, N., Weizhen, X. & Wang, Z. (2022a). Effects of sleep duration on neurocognitive development in early adolescents in the USA: A propensity score matched, longitudinal, observational study. *The Lancet Child & Adolescent Health*, 6(10), 705–712. https://doi.org/10.1016/S2352-4642(22)00188-2.

Yang, N., Liu, T.T. & Wang, Z. (2022b). Functional connectome mediates the association between sleep disturbance and mental health in preadolescence: A longitudinal mediation study, *Human Brain Mapping*, 43, 2041–2050. https://doi.org/10.1002/hbm.25772

Index[1]

[1] Note: Page numbers followed by 'n' refer to notes.

M. C. Nagel, R. Sharman, *Virtual Autism and Other Screen Disorders*, Palgrave Studies in Cyberpsychology, https://doi.org/10.1007/978-3-032-00803-9

FSC
www.fsc.org
MIX
Papier | Fördert
gute Waldnutzung
FSC® C083411

Kolibri 360 GmbH
Ferdinand-Jühlke-Straße 7
99095 Erfurt, Deutschland
produktsicherheit@kolibri360.de